Matthew Pennington
& Nicola Cradock

Do Ferment

Gut boosters and foods that fizz.

DO Book Co

For my Dad, whose kindness shaped my path and whose love of good food taught me its true worth. — **MP**

For my Mum and Dad, who have encouraged and believed in me every step of my journey. — **NC**

Published by
The Do Book Company 2025
Works in Progress Publishing Ltd
thedobook.co

A CIP catalogue record for this book is available from the British Library

ISBN 978-1-914168-52-9

10 9 8 7 6 5 4 3 2

To find out more about our company, books and authors, please visit **thedobook.co** or follow us **@dobookco**

5 per cent of our proceeds from the sale of this book is given to The DO Lectures to help it achieve its aim of making positive change: thedolectures.com

Cover designed by James Victore
Book designed and set by Ratiotype
Printed and bound in the EU by OZGraf on Munken, an FSC® certified paper
GPSR: productsafety@thedobook.co

MIX
Paper | Supporting responsible forestry
FSC® C163799

Contents

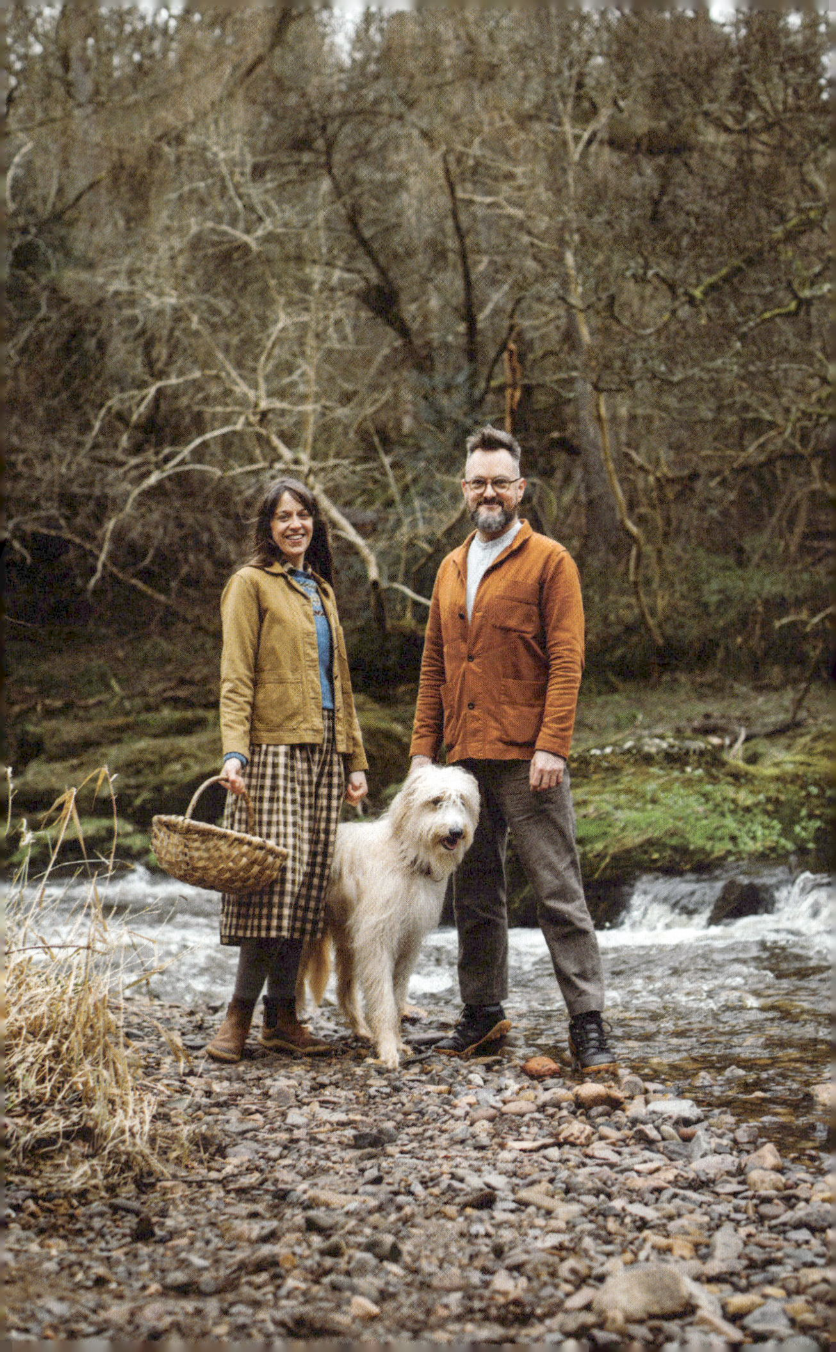

Prologue

It's early evening. There's warmth left in the sunlight, but it is cooler than usual for summer's end. We've left a hectic day behind us and are heading out for a walk to clear our minds and unwind. Our lurcher, Lint, trots alongside us, the air feels fresher and we've already begun to relax.

It's meadowsweet season, and our basket soon fills with clusters of frothy white flowers. We pick up on their sweet almond fragrance, sparking a familiar thought: how could we capture this moment? At once, we remember a punnet of plums loitering at home. Could these two humble ingredients be preserved and transformed into something delicious to enjoy long after the season passes?

Back at home, we add sea salt to the Jubilee plums, which have been ripening and softening. We've chosen salt over sugar this time because we have an inkling that this approach might work as well as it does with tomato fruits. We dip the whorls of fuzzy flowers into the pink and purple blush of the fruit in the jar, and they slowly submerge in the salty, sweet liquid that comes from within.

Over the coming days, we eagerly watch as bubbles begin to form. This tiny yet active and fizzy world looks magnificent when held up to the light. The meadowsweet blossoms in the syrupy juices look like seafoam, and the scent from the jar is now redolent with something *so close* to vanilla. We are awestruck and curious. A teaspoon in hand, we taste. Oh wow! The salt has doubled the natural sweetness, but fresh acidity is coming through, and the vanilla scent tastes closer to nutmeg now. How is this possible from just three simple ingredients? The answer: the magic of fermentation.

The glass lid is closed, and back up on the shelf it goes. Let's see what more time brings. So far, it already reminds us of our after-work meander. We look up and Lint is holding her lead in her mouth. Back out we go, this time to muse over how to use our new concoction.

Thinking about the long game, Matthew suggests a salt plum topping for rice pudding for later in autumn. With more immediacy, Nicola has her sights set on salt plum and meadowsweet margaritas for the evening...

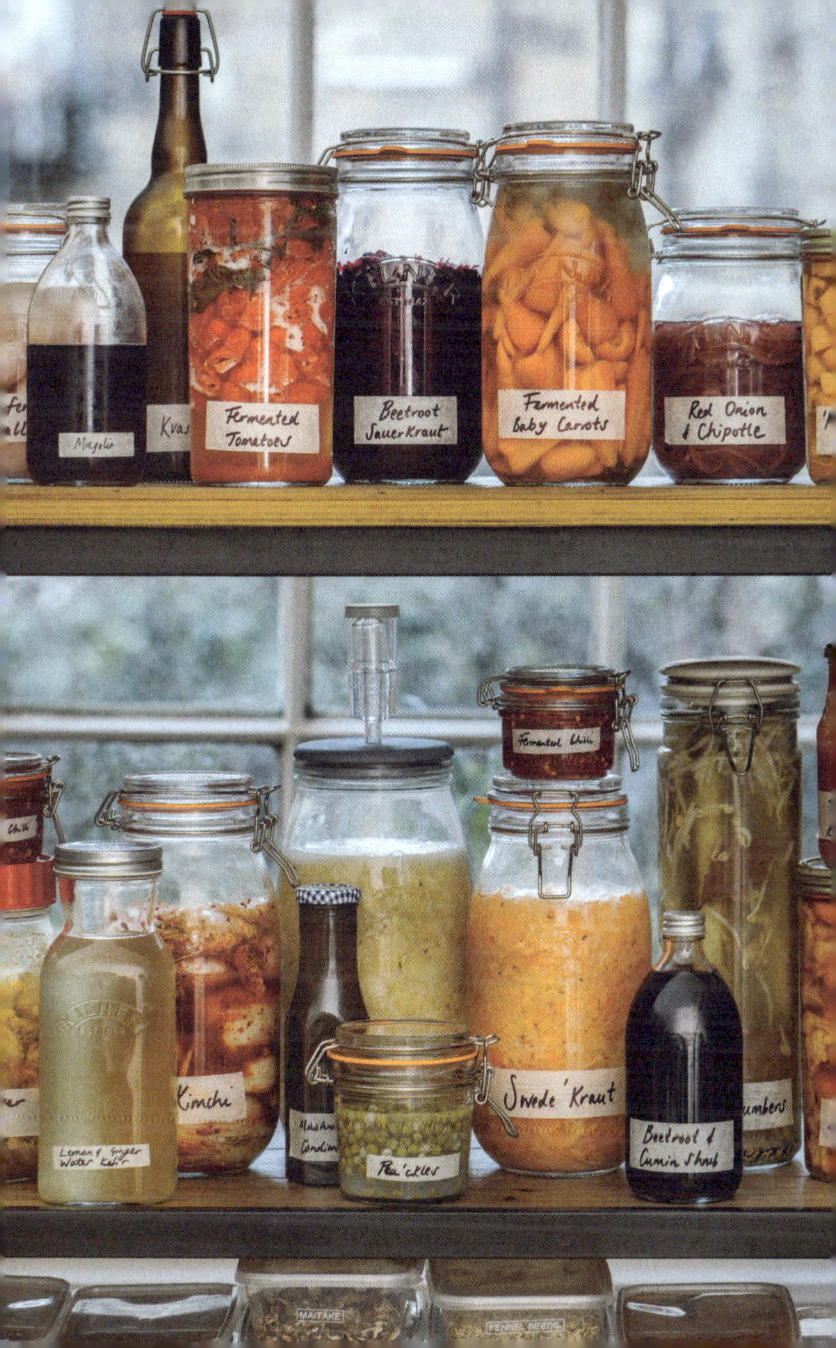
Fermented Tomatoes
Beetroot SauerKraut
Fermented Baby Carrots
Red Onion & Chipotle
Fermented Chilli
Kimchi
Swede 'Kraut
Beetroot & Cumin Shrub
Lemon & Ginger Water Kefir
Pea'ckles
MAITAKE
FENNEL SEEDS

Introduction

If you invite us over for a gathering, we're 'that couple', known for bringing a jar of fermented food or a bottle of homemade sparkling soda as a gift. Most often, it has reached peak deliciousness, and as the bottle pops, we're all in the moment, discovering something new together.

Our journey with fermentation is rooted in the kitchen garden restaurant we ran for 13 years — The Ethicurean, nestled in a Somerset orchard. There, we cooked and crafted drinks from native produce, foraged wild food and tumbled headfirst into the rabbit hole of fungi and soil health. We embraced all the peculiar pagan traditions — Midsummer, Apple Day and the deep-winter Wassail, where a raucous, cider-fuelled crowd would howl at the sky, hoping for a good apple crop the following year.

Guided by a simple ethos — working with what was available, as close to us as possible — we learned to preserve gluts in preparation for the hungry gap, be creative with ingredients and capture each season's bounty.

MATTHEW: My childhood was shaped by an outdoor upbringing, exploring nature through Cubs and Scouts. I was always drawn to the slow, hands-on processes of food, though I didn't yet have the language for it.

In 2009, I founded The Ethicurean, a natural continuation of that instinct to observe, learn and iterate. Fermentation became a key part of my cooking, a way to capture the living energy of an ingredient.

Over the years, I've become increasingly fascinated by the parallels between soil health, gut health and human wellbeing. Just as a thriving soil microbiome supports plant vitality, our own microbiome plays a crucial role in digestion, immunity and overall health. The more I explored these connections, the more fermentation made sense — not just as a means of preservation, but as a way to work with nature, harnessing its rhythms to create something deeply nourishing.

Nicola's arrival at the restaurant in 2017 sparked a new chapter. Together, we delved deeper, refining techniques and expanding our experiments. Fermentation became more than just a practice; it became a way of understanding the world, a lens through which we could explore everything from ancient traditions to modern science.

NICOLA: My connection to food began at an early age. I was raised on a fourth-generation family farm in Wiltshire, where the link between land, food and community was part of everyday life. One of my earliest memories is standing on hay bales piled onto a trailer while Dad drove the tractor through the fields. The whole family picked elderberries for Mum and Grandma to transform into wine, and I can still picture the demijohns bubbling away in the kitchen. Little did I know that what I was watching was fermentation!

When I joined The Ethicurean, I saw an opportunity to build on the foundations already in place — to create, experiment with, and explore the vast world of fermentation and wild drink making. I find particular joy in concocting wild sparkling sodas, fruit wines and bottled shrubs — tiny moments of calm amid the chaos of life. I love the rhythm of tending to kefir and always have a stash of thoughtfully made gifts ready for friends and family.

Over the years, we've deepened our curiosity, eager to understand not just fermentation itself but how it fits into the rhythm of daily life. There's something quietly satisfying about working side by side in the kitchen, a podcast playing in the background, hands gently processing ingredients — knowing that in days or weeks, something delicious will emerge. We still watch in awe, like children, as wild botanicals begin to fizz and come alive before our eyes.

In this book, we hope to share that sense of wonder, helping you craft your own ferments. It's about process, transformation and paying attention to what's right in front of us, and noticing the potential in seemingly ordinary things.

Let's see what we can make of them together.

Why we ferment

- We ferment for sheer enjoyment — to be alive, present and in the moment. It enables us to spend time with ourselves, to be distraction-free and scratch a creative itch.

- We ferment because we can take control of our health and wellbeing. We know that living food nourishes us. It nurtures the trillions of life forms that make up our human bodies, helping us feel at our best.

- We ferment because we can honour peak season ingredients and give them a long life. They taste delicious and are alive with a positivity we can feel.
- We ferment because we know a jar of something astonishing is waiting for us to share.

Food should heal, nourish and regenerate while fostering moments of fellowship and shared intimacy around the kitchen table. We both share a mission to challenge the status quo of convenience food: fast, overprocessed and empty. We aim to provide you with the tools to prepare minimally processed, nutrient-rich food that aligns with nature and is enjoyable to make and create.

On a personal level, we've both felt the benefits of microbially rich foods. In gradual steps, eating ferments over many months and years, we've noticed how positivity increased, sniffles and allergies retreated, and we have a newfound 'pep', eager to start each day.

Our fermentation journey

For over a decade, we've been immersed in a labyrinth of fermentation discovery, leaving very few corners of the subject unexplored. We had to close our beloved restaurant to pursue the next part of our culinary journey, but the knowledge we acquired there lives on.

The Ethicurean gave us a unique insight into the benefits of growing food according to no-dig and regenerative principles. The taste of vegetables grown this way is astonishing; food grown like this has far better flavour. And we understand that the soil can be seen as a stomach, much like ours, and thrives on careful input and tending.

We took those fruits, fungi and vegetables grown with natural craftsmanship and explored every possible fermentation technique we could research, creating everything from stunning lacto-ferments to fermented native barley. We built temperature and moisture-controlled cabinets to inoculate native grains like Hodmedod's Black Badger peas with Japanese 'white mould' koji spores to make miso. We aged that miso for two years, which was worth the wait. Steeped with native kelp at 60°C (140°F), it was about as moreish and nostalgic as you can imagine.

We even explored *deep breath* edible 'white mould' koji-spore-inoculated vegetable charcuterie. It is impractical but unforgettable, with a texture like cured beef bresaola and a taste reminiscent of rain on summer grass — a unique but lasting memory.

We understand that not everyone has time for such elaborate projects, but we are convinced that we all need to eat more of these 'alive' foods, little and often.

> **Perfection comes over time. Not at the start. Start where you are. But start.**
> DO Manifesto

We've fine-tuned our methods through years of research, experimenting, tasting and microbial testing and are genuinely excited to be sharing them with you. We've honed clever solutions that allow you and the microbes to be easily guided. If you need to go away for a few days and can't tend your microbial foods, just follow our steps and they will be alive and well upon your return.

We've learned some genuinely nifty ways to perfect homemade fermented foods. As we cook at home, we've also learned that simplicity is key. So, we have cherry-picked some simple fermenting principles from our experiences at The Ethicurean and from experimenting at home, which you can quickly master, each with limitless creative possibilities.

Research shows that regularly consuming a wide range of fermented foods or drinks is the key to a healthy diet, improving gut diversity and boosting immune health. We'll discuss great ferment pairings and inspiring ways to add them to your diet. Fermentation will ease into your life with minimal resistance and become a playground for flavour.

We will provide you with the 'aftercare' for your ferments and give you the confidence to overcome any hurdles in the fermentation process. We will guide you in building your living larder, which you can dip into across the weeks and months.

Fermentation is a craft that can bewitch, enchant and delight. Start small, be guided by our experience and enjoy the process.

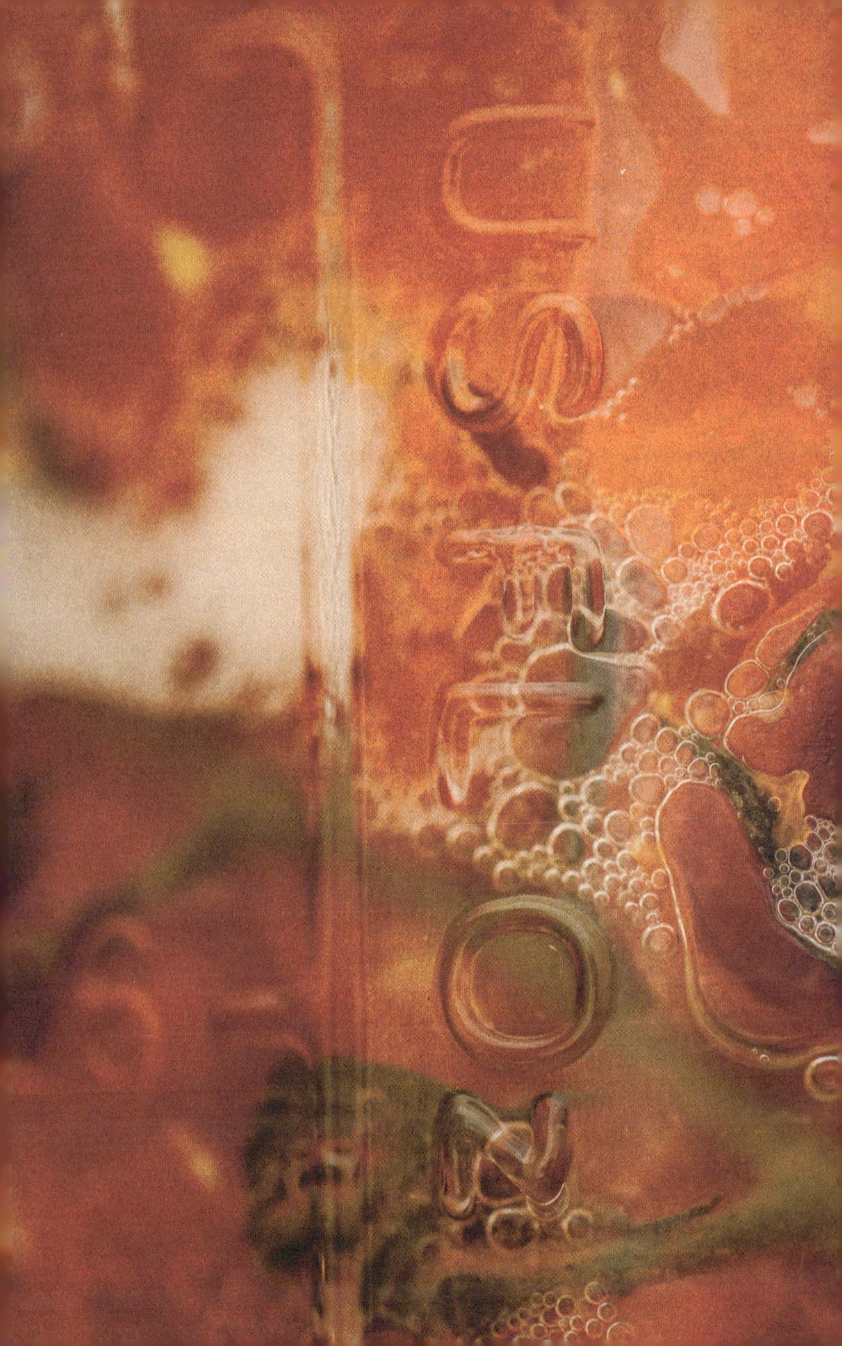

1

What is food and drink fermentation?

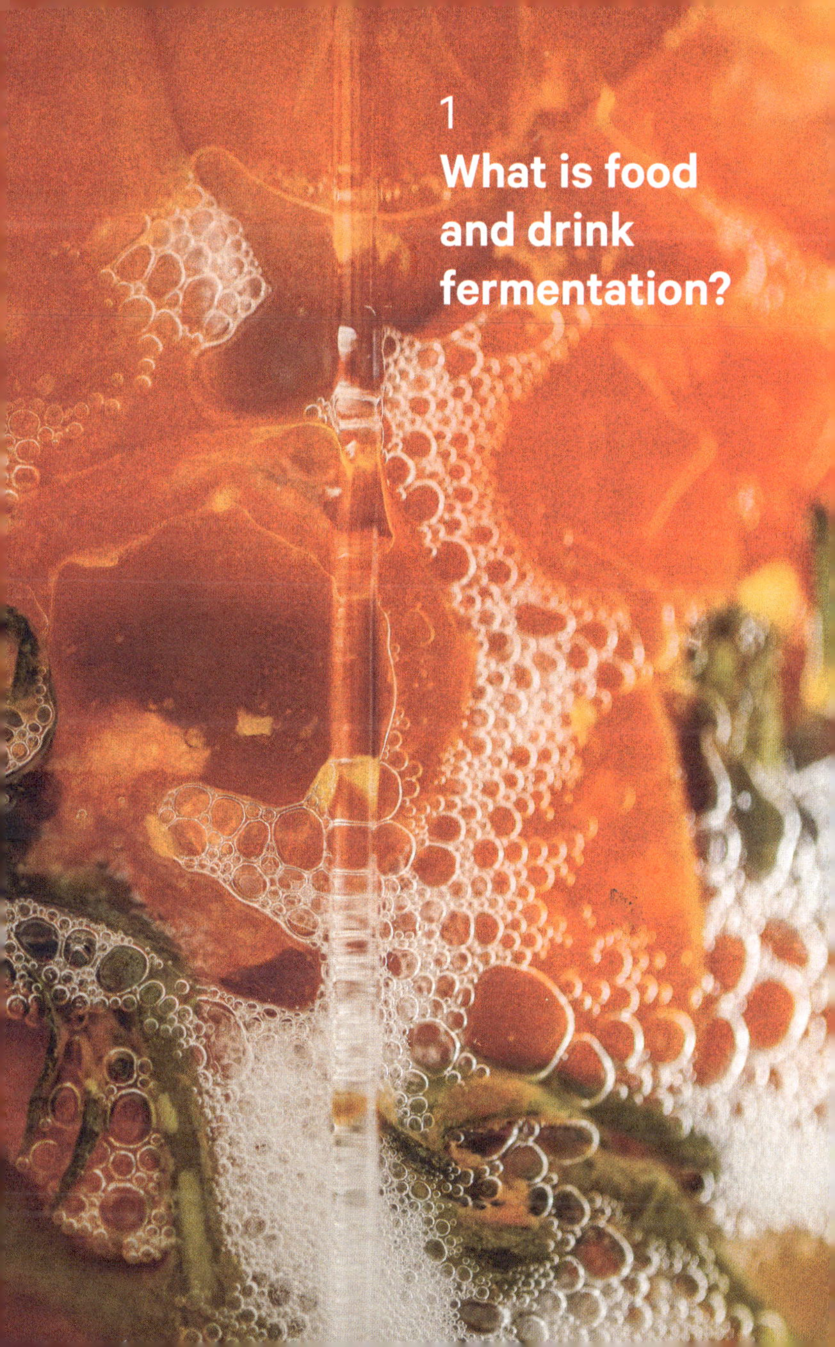

**Nature does not hurry,
yet everything is accomplished.**

Tao Te Ching

Fermentation is one of the oldest methods of food preservation humans have harnessed. Its exact origins remain unknown, but the beneficial bacteria, yeasts, fungi and microorganisms that drive fermentation are unimaginably ancient — they predate human civilisation by millennia.

We've all watched a bowl of fruit turn fuzzy and bloom in a kaleidoscope of intricate moulds. Our ancestors would have witnessed this, too. Yet occasionally, the outcome was different: the fruit slowly dried, moulds never took hold and it remained edible — transformed but preserved nonetheless. Likely, in this instance, sunlight and a constant warm breeze provided the ideal conditions to kick-start natural preservation.

Over time, humans discovered how to intentionally influence these processes. They observed that certain elements — like salt — played a crucial role. First mined and traded thousands of years ago, salt revolutionised food preservation. It draws moisture from fresh ingredients and can make a simple preserving brine. Using salt in preservation encourages beneficial microbes while suppressing harmful ones.

This simple yet profound discovery allowed early humans

to 'harvest' the power of microorganisms, creating a variety of preserved foods that were long lasting and delicious.

At its heart, fermentation is about leaving food in a state of happy stillness, creating an environment where microorganisms can thrive. These microbes break down sugars and carbohydrates, producing acids, alcohols or gases, which over time preserve food and transform its texture, flavour and nutritional profile.

Many of the foods and beverages we find irresistible owe their appeal to fermentation. Whether tangy, sharp or deeply savoury, fermented foods and drinks offer complexity and richness beyond their simple ingredients.

Fermentation pathways

There are three main 'pathways' of fermentation — lactic acid, alcoholic and acetic — creating many delicious foods or drinks.

- **Lactic acid fermentation** It is powered by lactic acid bacteria, which convert sugars and carbohydrates into lactic acid.

- **Alcoholic fermentation** Yeasts take the spotlight, transforming sugars into alcohol and carbon dioxide. This process gives us bread that rises, beers that fizz and wines that age gracefully.

- **Acetic fermentation** This type begins where alcoholic fermentation leaves off. Bacteria convert alcohol into acetic acid, the key component in vinegar.

Fermentation is not just about preservation — it's a tool for enhancing flavour and nutrition. For example, lactic acid fermentation produces vitamins (B and K), probiotics and enzymes that support digestion. It transforms a simple food into something extraordinary. Even foods not commonly considered 'fermented' — like chocolate, coffee and dried fruits — rely on fermentation during their production.

— **Chocolate** The journey of chocolate begins with fermentation. After cacao pods are harvested, the sticky white pulp surrounding the beans is left to ferment. Naturally occurring yeasts and bacteria break down the sugars, generating heat and acidity that develop the rich, complex flavours we associate with fine chocolate. Without this step, chocolate would taste flat and neutral.

— **Coffee** Fermentation is key to unlocking coffee's flavour. After coffee cherries are harvested, the mucilage — a sticky layer surrounding the beans — must be removed. This is achieved through fermentation, which enhances flavour notes ranging from fruity and floral to wine-like, depending on how the process is managed.

— **Dried fruits** Even sun-dried fruits like figs, dates and raisins undergo subtle fermentation. Wild yeasts and bacteria act on the sugars as the fruit dries, creating caramelised sweetness and complex flavour compounds.

— **Spices** Seed pods like vanilla and cardamom undergo fermentation during their curing process, a crucial step that develops the complex aromatic compounds that make them so prized. This transformation is mainly due to the breakdown and interaction of polyphenols, natural compounds abundant in spices.

Fermentation is a quiet yet transformative process, working below the surface to craft our most beloved foods. Whether carefully guided or left to nature, it preserves nutrients while creating layers of complexity and character. There is often a lively fizz to show for it.

Throughout this book, we will primarily harness the power of lactic acid fermentation (with a nod to acetic fermentation) to create preserved food bursting with flavour, texture and nutritional goodness. You'll learn how to transform simple ingredients into vibrant, living, gut-boosting foods by cultivating the ideal conditions for beneficial microbes to thrive.

Flavour: The Vinegar Tasters

In the story of *The Vinegar Tasters*, retold by Benjamin Hoff in *The Tao of Pooh*, three men taste vinegar, each reacting differently — perceiving it as sour, bitter or sweet — reflecting their unique worldviews. Yet despite their differing interpretations, the vinegar itself remains the same, reminding us that our individual flavour experiences are profoundly personal and shaped by culture, memory and tastes.

Ferments, too, invite this variety of responses. To one person, a tangy sauerkraut might be enjoyably sharp; to another, it might seem too bold or unusual. Yet when we approach ferments with curiosity and an open mind, we often discover something extraordinary: a shared feeling that these foods, with their layers of complexity, are delicious in a way that transcends personal preference.

Just as the vinegar doesn't change, but our perception of it does, ferments remain constant in transforming simple ingredients into something more significant. The beauty of this process lies in creating food you enjoy and exploring flavours that connect us to an ancient tradition and each other.

Not every ferment will taste the same to everyone, but the journey of tasting, observing and understanding is one we all share. In that sense, ferments become more than just food; they bridge our tastes and a collective experience of discovery.

Gut health: a path to wellbeing

The book *Immune* by Philipp Dettmer opened our eyes to how astonishingly complex our biological systems are. The human body isn't just 'us'; we're ecosystems, home to trillions of microbes that keep us alive and healthy.

This glimpse into our complexity is humbling. Health isn't a linear equation, and there's no one-size-fits-all solution; we are, after all, a unique package of those trillions of microbes, each of us with differing needs. However, one simple and impactful step to improving gut health is gradually incorporating more fermented foods into your daily life. By doing so, you'll support your gut with beneficial microbes while shifting towards a diet rooted in fresh, seasonal and delicious ingredients.

> **The diversity of our gut bacteria is a reflection of the diversity of our diet and lifestyle.**
> Tim Spector

Of course, other factors are at play in supporting your wellbeing, such as nutritional balance, physical movement and exercise, sleep quality, stress and exposure to toxins (industrial and environmental). Still, as we will explore, food underpins your resilience in these areas. When we make choices about what we eat, we alter how we think and feel and, therefore, achieve wellness.

The beauty of fermented foods lies in their versatility. Whether it's a spoonful of sauerkraut, a sip of kvass, or a glug of milk kefir, each small addition contributes to building a healthier, more balanced approach to eating while maintaining the equilibrium of your gut flora. Throughout this book, we'll guide you on introducing these foods into your weekly routine, showing you how to create, enjoy and benefit from them step by step.

This isn't about a dramatic overhaul or chasing dietary perfection. It's about making small, steady changes that naturally lead you away from ultra-processed foods and towards vibrant, nourishing choices. The goal is to inspire curiosity, encourage experimentation and help you take those first strides towards a lifestyle enriched by fermented foods.

While scientific research continues to explore the intricacies of gut health, incorporating fermented foods into your daily diet has undeniable benefits. These foods are rich in live cultures, enzymes and bioavailable nutrients that can support digestion, encourage microbial diversity and strengthen your gut barrier.

Fermented vegetables also come with a giant bonus: they enhance the fibre content of your meals. Vegetable ferments are typically made with non-starchy vegetables such as alliums, brassicas and their cruciferous offspring, cucurbits, capsicums, mustards, fungi and nightshades — onions, kales, cucumbers, peppers, cabbage, leafy greens, mushrooms and tomatoes — all the vegetable types that contain a high fibre-to-carbohydrate ratio. Fibre is vital for a healthy gut. It helps keep things moving and aids digestion. Fibre also carries nutrients deeper into the gut, where our unique bacterial colonies thrive.

Fermented produce is unique because the fermentation process makes the fibre more accessible and thus easier for your gut microbes to break down. This means that your gut gets extra support from the very microbes that help you digest the fibre in the first place.

On your path to improving wellbeing, we encourage you to explore, observe and think more about your consumption. Gut health is about balance, diversity and curiosity. It's about making choices that move you towards feeling good — thoughtful decisions about what you eat and which foods you can easily substitute in place of detrimental ones.

Fermentation is a practical and delicious way to adopt a healthier mindset. By making and consuming fermented foods, you add beneficial microbes to your diet and choose real, nourishing ingredients.

There's something inherently rewarding about sourcing the best vegetables, experimenting with flavours, embracing the nutritional power of spices, and tasting the results of your efforts.

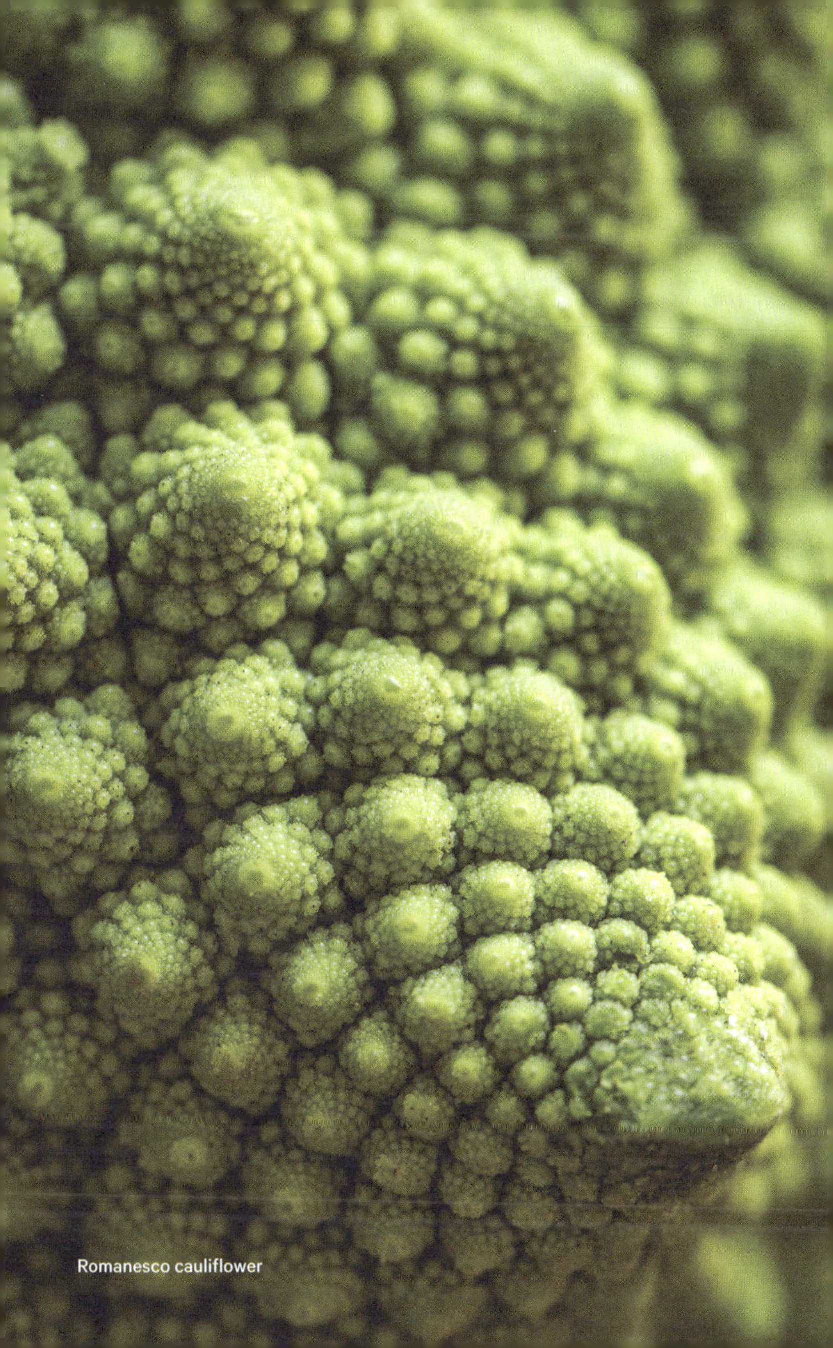

Romanesco cauliflower

Lactobacillus

We begin this journey into food fermentation by appreciating the star of the show: lactobacillus. Please be upstanding for this genuinely astonishing microbe.

This beneficial bacterium transforms simple ingredients — like vegetables, milk and grains — into delicious, tangy and probiotic-rich foods. As it thrives, it creates a naturally acidic environment that preserves food and keeps out harmful bacteria.

What makes lactobacillus extraordinary is its versatility and resilience. You'll find it in everything from sauerkraut and yoghurt to sourdough bread. It's also a resident in our digestive systems, where it plays a vital role in maintaining gut health and balance. Lactobacillus thrives in oxygen-free environments, like those created during fermentation, and flourishes particularly well in specific salt concentrations — a topic we'll explore later.

Lactobacillus takes centre stage during vegetable fermentation in a process called 'microbial succession'. Initially, various microorganisms interact with the food, but lactobacillus quickly dominates. It produces lactic acid, which lowers the pH and creates an environment hostile to spoilage microbes. Over several weeks, differing strains of lactobacillus will thrive, digest their food and then fall back, full but sleepy, for the next strain. This is why we describe it as a microbial succession.

Temperature plays a key role in the speed of this process, with cooler conditions leading to slower but often more complex ferments. For example, at 12°C (54°F), the fermentation process might take around four weeks. At 18°C (64°F), the process may speed up to three weeks. As a side note, at around 20°C (68°F) and upwards, there are strains of lactobacillus that produce some of the funkier, more, how should we say, 'farmyard-like' smells. You may be entirely okay with this, but as a preference, we aim to ferment from 10–18°C (50–64°F). Understandably, you may be reading this from a warmer country and might have to make more effort to find a cool cupboard or larder to ferment to this temperature. Modifying a dedicated fridge to run at 10–14°C (50–57°F) might be worth considering in exceptional circumstances. This temperature range does create some incredible results and, as Harold McGee explains in *On Food and Cooking*, different lactobacillus strains thrive at various fermentation stages:

— **Early stages:** 1–2 weeks at 21°C (70°F) or 2–3 weeks at 12°C (54°F). Strains like *Lactobacillus plantarum* and *Lactobacillus brevis* dominate, kick-starting the fermentation by rapidly producing lactic acid and lowering the pH.

— **Later stages:** 2–4 weeks at 21°C (70°F) or 3–5 weeks at 12°C (54°F). As acidity increases and pH drops further, strains such as *Lactobacillus sakei* and *Lactobacillus mesenteroides* take over, ensuring a robust and stable fermentation environment.

But lactobacillus doesn't stop at preservation. It enriches food by producing vitamins like B12 and K and enzymes that help break down nutrients, making them easier for us to digest. Thanks to this tiny powerhouse, you're not just preserving food — you're transforming it into something more nutritious, flavourful and beneficial for your gut health, bone density and nervous system function.

Salt

For thousands of years, salt didn't just season food; it preserved, protected and extended its life far beyond the limits of its natural decay.

Salt is the bedrock of flavour. Salt allows us to produce lacto-fermented vegetables or hasten milk storage in aged cheese. Nearly every seasoning humans have invented—spices, pastes or marinades—owes its existence to salt. Yet its significance extends beyond the culinary. Sodium chloride, NaCl, is life itself. It is essential to life because it helps regulate the balance of fluids in all living organisms. It is key in hydration, nerve transmission and cellular function. Without salt, the world as we know it would cease to exist.

> **Rice without salt is like life without laughter.**
> Iain Pennington

Imagine tasting seawater for the first time. Bitter, briny and oddly comforting. It speaks of something ancient, something elemental. Over millennia, rain chiselled away at unyielding mountains, freeing salt crystals trapped in stone and carrying them to the sea. Coastal foragers cooked their meals in seawater, unaware they were witnessing the beginnings of preservation.

The ancient Egyptians are thought to be the first to have industrialised salt. They coaxed crystals from seawater at coastal evaporation sites using nothing but the sun's heat. This ingenuity spread across the globe, inspiring other methods: brine pits, salt mines and, in modern times, chemical production. Yet, in every era, salt remained more than a mineral. It is worth its weight in gold.

During the Anglo-Saxon era, the phrase 'put salt on it'

likely rang out in the bustling *-wich* (salt pit) towns of England — Nantwich, Northwich, Middlewich and York (Jorvic). Far from the sea, these towns thrived on their brine pits and salt mines. They weren't just places of trade but hubs of food preservers with their wares. Salt underpinned entire economies, creating connections within communities and kitchens.

In fermentation, salt is the silent partner in food transformation. Sprinkle it on vegetables and water weeps from their cells. This protective brine creates a shield that wards off harmful bacteria while nurturing the microbes we seek to encourage.

Salt is the constant in our quest for preservation, a cornerstone of flavour and the alchemical force that makes fermentation possible. To work with salt is to join a lineage of preservers, cooks, foragers and artisans who understood its power and value.

Two per cent

Traditionally, cookbooks follow the same format: ingredients weighed out and listed in order of use. However, as working cooks, we use 'percentage of the whole' more often. Recipes written as a 'percentage of the whole' apply very well to cake baking and pastry work, but especially to the fermenting of food.

The salt concentration in a ferment matters deeply — too little and the wrong microbes flourish; too much and fermentation grinds to a halt. Through observation, experimentation and microbial testing, we found the sweet spot for the specific types of lactobacillus we wanted to see thrive in our ferments.

While researching old fermentation recipes, we noticed they often used a pinch, a punch, a cup and other vague measurements, presumably from a time without scales to measure with. Thankfully, with the metric system and inexpensive scales now commonplace, the guesswork can be banished, and we can celebrate consistency in cooking.

Bakers and pastry chefs have long used percentages in commercial kitchens so we adapted this ideology and applied it to understanding fermentation. Scientific? Perhaps, but it is very easy to grasp and allows you the freedom to ferment random amounts of vegetables, which is how you'll often find them in a veg box or harvested in peak season.

Using a percentage of salt (usually 2%) for fermentation recipes ensures consistency across batches because you maintain a precise balance of salt to ingredients, regardless of batch size. It promotes ideal microbial growth, fostering beneficial lactic acid bacteria while inhibiting harmful pathogens, resulting in safe and reliable ferments.

Vegetable weight	Salt required
500g	10g
750g	15g
1kg	20g
1.25kg	25g
1.5kg	30g

2% salt calculation: vegetable weight × 0.02, e.g. 1,350g × 0.02 = 27g salt required.

This approach prevents over-salting, ensuring the final product isn't unpalatable. It also optimises brine formation by drawing water out of the ingredients through osmosis, creating the perfect environment for fermentation. Since vegetables vary in water content and density, calculating salt as a percentage ensures the recipe adapts to these differences, delivering consistent results. (Handy fact: one millilitre of water weighs one gram.)

Using a percentage of salt supports long-term preservation by slowing fermentation, allowing complex flavours to develop while keeping the ferment safe and stable. It improves texture by helping vegetables retain their crunch.

This method makes scaling recipes easy for a single jar or a large batch while adhering to the same ratio. The practice is grounded in tradition and science, aligning with tested microbial thresholds for safe food production.

Throughout this book, recipes will jump in and out of conventional ingredients listings. In some cases, where we have two-part recipes (lime-fermented shallots and zero-waste fermented lime 'pickle'), we add weights because we call for 500g (1lb 2oz) of shallots and 10 limes, giving you a 1kg (2lb 4oz) jar of shallots and a 500g (1lb 2oz) jar of lime pickle.

Imperial measurements

Now, the '2 per cent rule' doesn't work so well if you're used to imperial measurements. But we've done the maths for you and provided some conversions (see overleaf) as a guide, rounded for ease. While they'll get you close to a 2% salt concentration, they aren't exact. But that's okay, you can tweak them as you get further into your fermentation journey.

If you're keen to refine your craft, we recommend investing in a digital kitchen scale with a unit-switching function. Just like a pH meter (see page 46), it makes life easier and gives you the confidence to accurately salt your ferments. A small step, but one that makes a big difference.

Metric to imperial conversions

Vegetable weight metric	**2% salt required** metric	**Vegetable weight** imperial	**2% salt required** imperial
500g	10g	approx. 1lb 2oz	2 tsp*
750g	15g	approx. 1lb 10oz	3 tsp
1kg	20g	approx. 2lb 4oz	4 tsp
1.25kg	25g	approx. 2lb 12oz	5 tsp
1.5kg	30g	approx. 3lb 3oz	6 tsp

*(Assuming 1 teaspoon of fine salt = 5g)

So, for every approx. 1lb of veg, you need just under 2 tsp of salt.

Why we insist on natural salts in fermentation

Many people ask us why we don't use table salt, especially when it comes to fermentation. We've always insisted on using natural salts in our cooking and never looked back. This decision is based on our belief that the quality of the ingredients we choose significantly impacts the flavour and health benefits and the overall integrity of the food we prepare. After all, we are going to eat it. Our food becomes us.

Unlike their processed counterparts, natural salts offer a depth of taste and essential minerals that table salt cannot.

There are many reasons for this, but they are simple when you break them down. Often highly refined, table salt lacks essential trace minerals like magnesium, potassium and calcium, which are crucial for both the flavour and the texture of our ferments. It is imperative when making pickles or other fermenting vegetables where the crunch is just as vital as the taste. Additives such as anti-caking agents and iodine can disrupt microbial activity, leading to inconsistent results and interfering with the growth of beneficial bacteria. The lack of calcium can affect the texture of fermented vegetables, causing them to lose their crunch. Additionally, table salt's sharp, metallic taste can overpower the subtle flavours developed during fermentation. Overuse of table salt can also contribute to health issues like hypertension, as it offers little nutritional value compared to natural salts.

The type of natural salt used — sea salt or rock salt — can influence the ferment's final flavour, texture and mineral content. Here's a few suggestions depending on where you are in the world.

Halen Môn is a widely available Welsh artisan sea salt, valued for its purity, rich mineral content and subtly sweet flavour. However, there's a whole world of natural salts to explore. You might experiment with other sea salts like Maldon, sel gris, fleur de sel, or Scottish Blackthorn salt, each offering unique textures and mineral profiles. Rock salts, formed deep underground, tend to be less processed and more raw in character. Himalayan pink salt and Redmond Real Salt from Utah all bring distinct flavours and trace minerals to your ferments, subtly shaping their final taste and texture.

Tannins and calcium chloride

Some additions are necessary to maintain crispness and texture when fermenting softer vegetables like cucumbers and squash. To maintain the bite of these soft vegetables, you can either use natural tannins or calcium chloride. Many plants contain tannin, and these have been used in fermenting for centuries. Here are some of our favourite tannin-rich plants to use when fermenting soft vegetables:

- Oak leaves
- Bay leaves
- Black tea leaves
- Horseradish leaves
- Cherry leaves
- Grape vine leaves

If none of these are available to you, use food-grade calcium chloride salt—sometimes branded as 'Pickle Crisp'. You only need a tiny amount: 0.01% or 1g (⅕ tsp) per litre (4 cups).

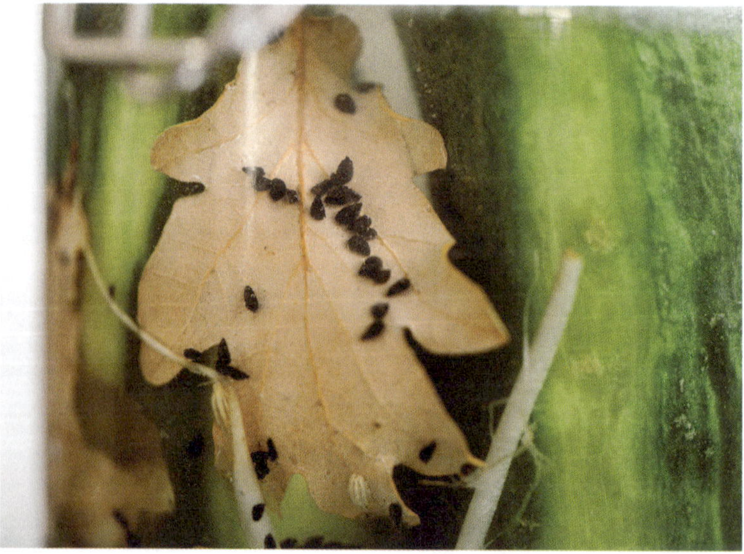

Spices: adding another dimension

Spices are a cornerstone of both flavour and health. They are rich in polyphenols, offering antioxidant and anti-inflammatory benefits that support overall wellness. So incorporating spices, especially those enriched through fermentation, is a straightforward win.

Enzymes and microorganisms act on these compounds during fermentation, breaking them into smaller, more volatile molecules that unlock complex, layered flavours. Fermentation doesn't just intensify these aromas; it opens them up over a much longer (and less intense) time frame, sometimes a minute or more.

We invite you to join us in an inspiration exercise. Grab a jar of spice seeds from your cupboard — you might reach for seeds like allspice, celery, cardamom, caraway, ajwain, clove, coriander, cumin, aniseed, fennel, juniper, lovage, mustard seed, nigella seed, peppercorn, star anise or sumac. Open the jar and let the scent fill the air — the volatile compounds of the spice quickly dash for atmospheric freedom, creating heady aromas. As you acclimatise to these scents, take a deeper breath and get closer to the jar. At this point, you might notice a memory surfacing — perhaps of a specific time of year, a place, or a person who cooked for you. These memories often evoke distinct feelings, whether positive or aversive.

Take a bite of your chosen spice seed and focus on what unfolds over the next few moments. In its dried state, the spice will rapidly reveal its flavours and effects on your tongue, and a sensory pop from the plant's defence compounds, within a few seconds. Plants develop these polyphenol-rich compounds as a defence mechanism against oxidative stress, UV damage and pests — a strategy honed over millennia of sunlight and heat in tropical and subtropical regions where many spices originate.

Given their profound nutritional benefits, spices deserve a special focus, especially when it comes to food fermentation. It's utterly fascinating and something we can explore again once you have a finished ferment.

Fermented foods: living and thriving

In fermentation, you create the conditions for beneficial bacteria, yeasts and enzymes to thrive. From this point on, think of yourself as a 'microbe farmer'. Your role is simply to guide the process, provide the right conditions and let these tiny organisms do the hard work.

With just a little care, some salt and a few simple kitchen tools, those microbes will transform your ingredients into vibrant, nutrient-rich food and drinks bursting with flavour. Whether it's crunchy fermented vegetables, more-ish condiments, or gut-boosting beverages, this preservation method unlocks an entire realm of possibilities.

Throughout this book, we'll show you how easy it is to bring fermentation into your kitchen. It requires minimal equipment, uses techniques at your fingertips and delivers transformative benefits for your health and mindset. You're about to master an age-old culinary craft that's as rewarding to practise as the results are delicious to eat. And we have every confidence in you.

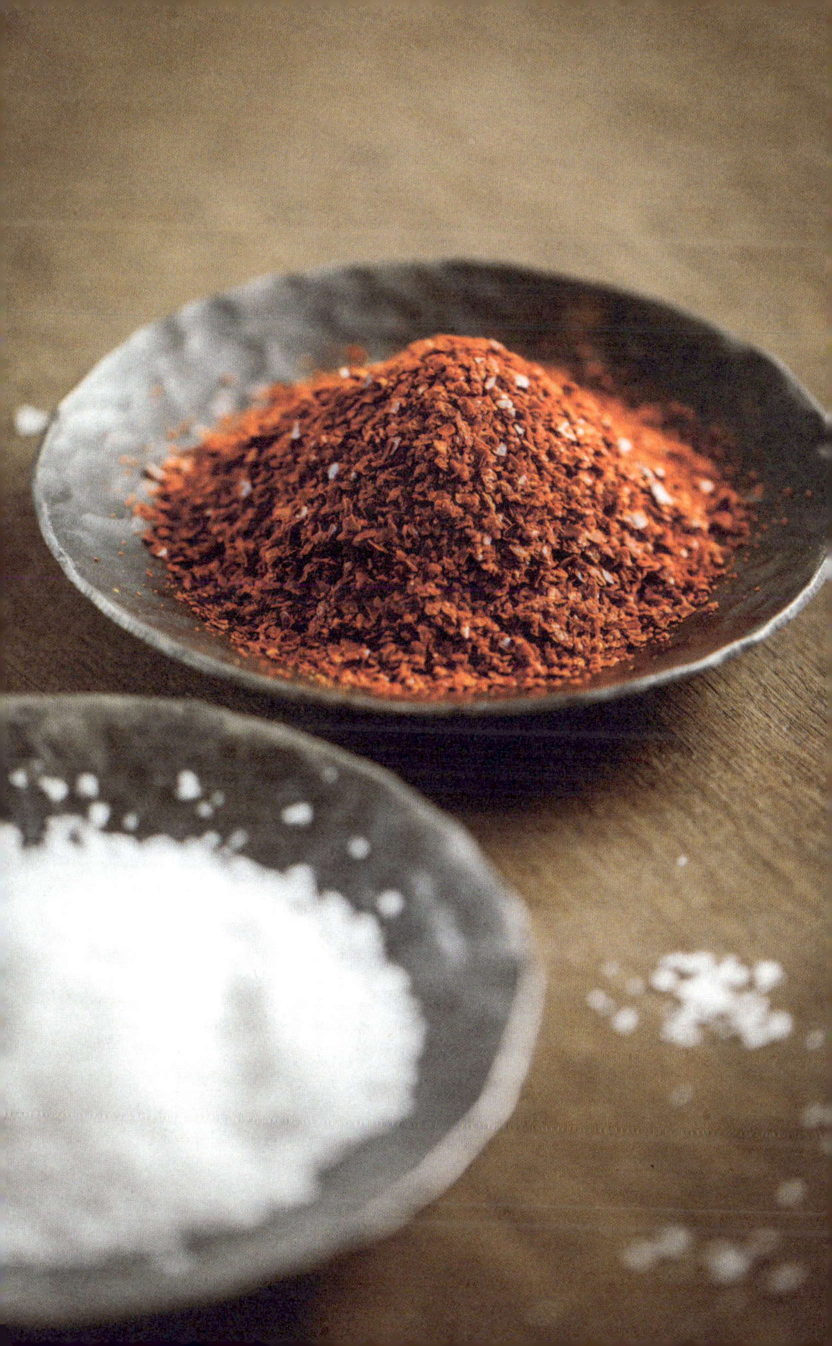

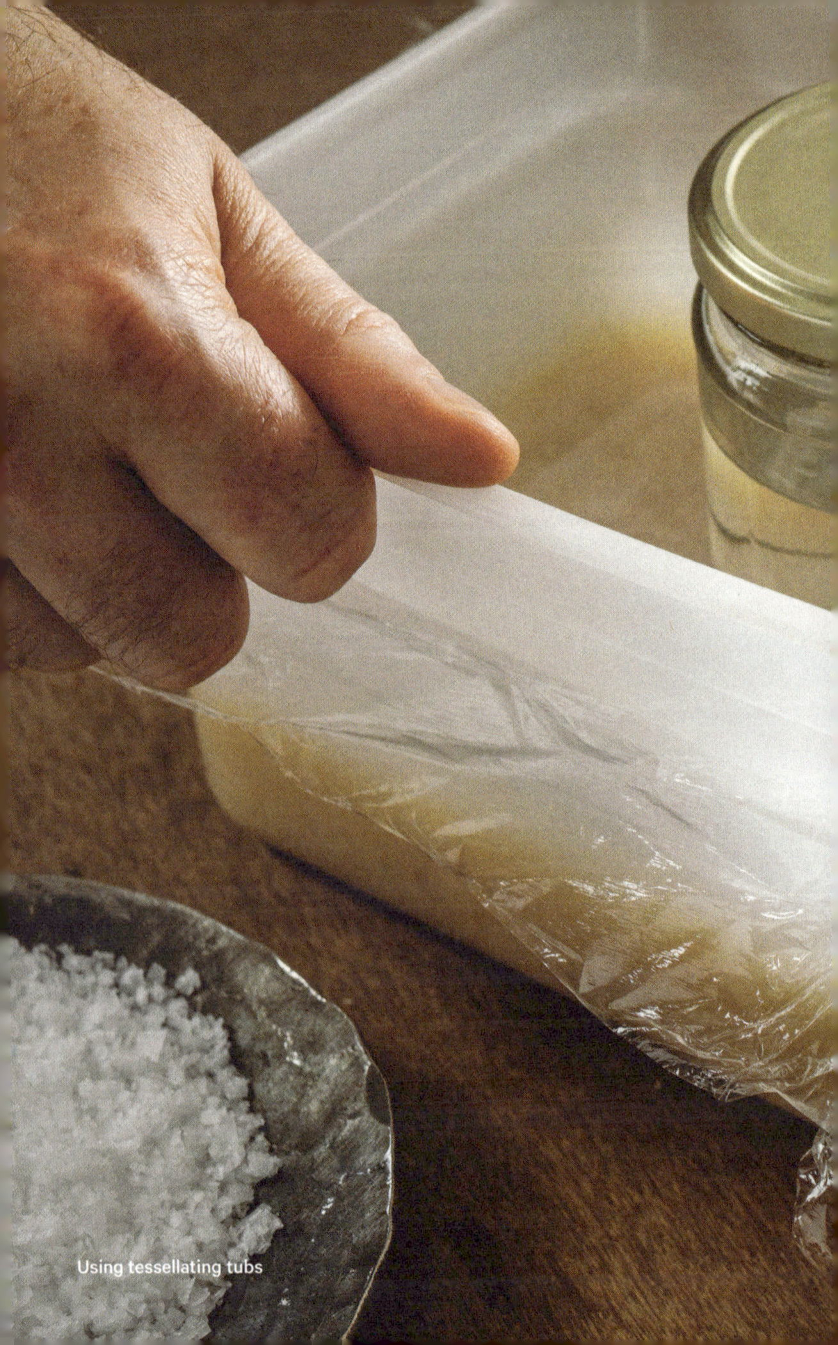

Using tessellating tubs

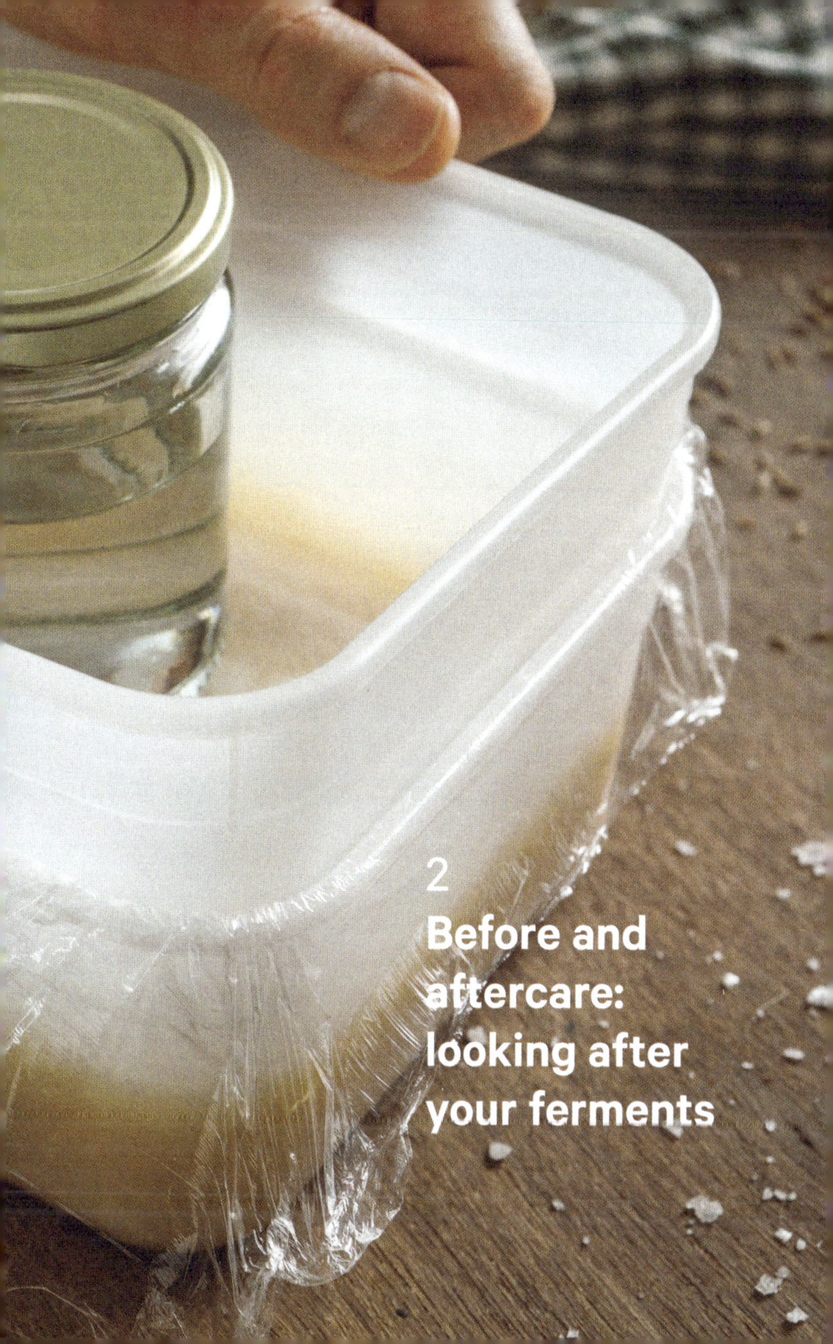

2
Before and aftercare: looking after your ferments

Before you let off some steam by shredding and massaging a cabbage, let's focus on the most crucial aspect of fermentation: before and aftercare. Understanding the before and aftercare of your fermentation projects is essential for achieving success.

To ensure successful fermentation, you'll need the following: your choice of fruits or vegetables, salt, an anaerobic (oxygen-free) environment and a comfortable temperature range. That's all there is to it.

Fresh fruit and vegetables

Seek out in-peak-season fruit and vegetables, which offer the best prices and optimal freshness. Whenever possible, use the freshest-looking produce and avoid anything limp or mouldy. Revive wilting vegetables by soaking them in cold water to restore their crispness before use.

All vegetables should be cleaned of soil sources. Take particular care with rhizomes such as ginger and turmeric, their unusual shape often harbours soil residue. It's best to peel vegetables before fermenting if they're non-organic or too soily. Well-washed, organic veg can have the peel left on.

Environment

Your ferment is a living thing — think of it as a pet that needs simple, occasional care:

- **Temperature:** Keep your ferment at a comfortable range, ideally 10–18°C (50–64°F). Too hot, and it may spoil; too cold, and it will ferment very slowly.

- **Anaerobic environment:** Ensure the vegetables are fully submerged in their brine to keep oxygen out and prevent unwanted moulds or yeasts. Check for submersion every couple of days. If needed, empty and repack your jar to rotate the contents.

- **Watch for activity:** Within a day or two, bubbles will form as fermentation begins. That's a good sign! That is the digestion gas, carbon dioxide. As the weeks progress, these bubbles will slow. Observing the bubbles is the easiest way to see how far along a ferment is.

An ideal ferment takes at least three weeks at the temperature we recommend. Many online sources suggest 3–5 days, which is not long enough for the slow-digesting microbes. Be patient. Refrigerating a ferment that has had such a short time to ferment could lead to a build up of pressure which may cause the vessel to break, and increase the risk of forming moulds that will eat the undigested, and not yet fully fermented veg.

Lactobacillus loves to be left for 3–4 weeks and will be very stable and developed in flavour and acidity at the end of this time. So be patient, watch the bubbles slow, and taste or test for acidity (see page 46). Ferments will develop tangy, fresh or sour notes over time.

They are comparable to basic kinds of vinegar in acidity. Trust your senses and taste to monitor progress.

Water

In the UK, tap water is generally treated with chlorine, which can negatively affect fermentation by killing the good bacteria essential for the process. To avoid this, boil your water first and let it cool to room temperature. Alternatively, you can use filtered water if you have access to it.

Hygiene

It's completely understandable to have some initial fears about the safety of fermentation, especially if you're familiar with the risks that can come with traditional preservation methods, like the potential for botulism.*
Many people think that the same dangers could arise with lacto-fermentation, but by the end of this book, you'll see that two factors, salt and acidity, make this preservation method the safest of them all.

Lacto-fermentation doesn't rely on creating a sterile environment or eliminating all microbes, as traditional methods do. Instead, it uses beneficial bacteria—primarily

---

* Botulism is caused by *clostridium botulinum*, which thrives in low-oxygen, low-acid environments—like improperly canned or preserved foods. When it grows, it releases a toxin in the form of a bacterium spore so potent that even tiny amounts can cause serious illness. But don't worry: this bacterium doesn't stand a chance in the acidic and salty conditions of lacto-fermentation. Think of it this way: botulism is a rare and dangerous intruder that needs just the right conditions to cause harm. Thankfully, lacto-fermentation creates the opposite environment, making it one of the safest ways to preserve food at home.

lactobacillus — to create a natural, acidic environment where only safe microbes can thrive. This self-regulating process is far more straightforward and carries a much lower risk than techniques that depend on intensive sterilisation or high temperatures.

As with all good kitchen practices, we recommend that utensils, pots, tubs, jam jars and clip-top jars be washed in hot, soapy water and rinsed clean. You don't need to sterilise your jars as salt is highly anti-pathogenic. Our preference is for wooden chopping boards.

Equipment

Having the right equipment makes fermentation straightforward. We recommend the below as basic kit, some of which you'll likely already have in your kitchen:

— **Digital scales:** For precise weighing of your ingredients (in 1g increments).

— **Tessellating tubs:** Straightforward, inexpensive and effective (see page 44 and image page 38–39).

— **Fermentation vessels:** A selection of jars, some with screw caps, some with clip tops. We mostly use 1 litre Kilner (Mason) jars.

— **Cling film:** Used directly on the surface of the ferment to act as a barrier to yeasts and moulds.

— **Thermometer:** To get a quick and accurate reading of the environment in which a ferment is living, to gauge if it requires moving somewhere cooler / warmer.

— **Muslin cloths or tea towels:** These act as a cover to stop insects getting to your ferments. You'll need string or an elastic band to secure them.

— **Labels:** A way of labelling your ferments with the date started, salt percentage, flavour / spices used etc. Masking tape and a pen work fine for this.

— **Vegetable peeler:** Perfect for finely shredding cabbage for sauerkrauts.

— **Sieve and funnel:** Useful equipment, particularly when making/bottling fermented condiments and drinks.

Tessellating 'ice cream' tubs

There are many options for containers to ferment food in, including some brilliant airtight solutions, such as E-Jen containers and Kilner jars with airlocks and weights. There are also natural, lead-free ceramics that are beautifully handmade for the task.

During our restaurant days we wanted a fermented element on every dish we served. It was a tall task, meaning ten or more ferments were bubbling each week — across a month, it would number 40. So, working at scale, we had to be creative and slowly build our collection of ready-made fermentation vessels, while also reaching for something inexpensive.

You might have spotted that in every commercial kitchen worldwide, food is stored in 2 litre (68fl oz) and 4 litre (135fl oz) food-grade tubs with plastic lids. Ice cream containers. These have a particular characteristic: when stacked, they have a very close tessellation in that they fit together with no gaps. We noticed that if you put a sauerkraut in the bottom tub, leave it unlidded and place an identical tub on top, the liquid layer keeps the ferment submerged; almost none of the ferment is exposed to air and the gases can escape. Then, with a lidded jam jar filled with water acting as a weight, the liquid layer is height adjustable to ensure an air-free environment. Adding a layer of cling film between the two tubs creates a secondary dust screen securing the ferment even further. See image on page 38–39 for a visual guide.

The quality of the ferments we produced in this set-up levelled up remarkably because we could achieve the three to four weeks at 10–18°C (50–64°F), prevent spoilage from yeasts and moulds, and they required very little daily double-checking. At home, such a set-up can allow you to leave ferments for a week without worrying if they'll survive.

In a perfect system, we recommend fermenting in glass or food-grade ceramic containers, but don't let expenses stop you from accessing the benefits of eating fermented food. Using tessellating food-grade tubs can be a quick, readily available option. Save up ice cream tubs to re-use — they just need to be the identical size and shape. Alternatively, nip into a restaurant near you and befriend the chef, ask for a couple of tubs and share your ferments with them.

Additional equipment which you could invest in if you'd like to take your fermentation to the next level:

- **Weights:** Glass or ceramic. To keep ingredients submerged below brine level.

- **Jar with airlock:** Specially designed to allow the gas to escape from a ferment, avoiding the need to 'burp' your creations.

- **Mandoline:** The next step up from your vegetable peeler in shredding vegetables finely for sauerkrauts, it will allow you to take on larger amounts in a short space of time. Use with caution, they're incredibly sharp.

- **pH meter:** A handheld home pH meter is a device used to measure the acidity of a solution. Immerse the probe in your ferment and it displays from 0 (very acidic) to 14 (very alkaline), with 7 being neutral. Using a pH meter allows for quick, accurate readings and helps maintain the proper balance needed for fermentation of sub 4.5.

pH / acidity

To expand, pH measures how acidic or alkaline a substance is on a scale of 0 to 14, with lower values indicating higher acidity. Acidity (low pH 3.0–4.0) in fermentation is critical because it creates an environment that inhibits harmful bacteria and promotes the growth of beneficial microbes like lactic acid bacteria (LAB). A pH below 4.5 is ideal for most ferments, and testing can confirm that long-term storage is possible. You can also test ferments that have been stored for months to check that they are still below 4.5.

It doesn't take long to train the palate and nose to recognise a safe level of acidity. Ferments should be acidic, much like a basic vinegar you have at home, so taste vinegar for comparison and learn to recognise acidity levels. A malt vinegar of 5% acidity will have a pH of about 2.8. Alternatively, a handheld pH meter is a valuable yet inexpensive piece of equipment for the home and professional fermenter.

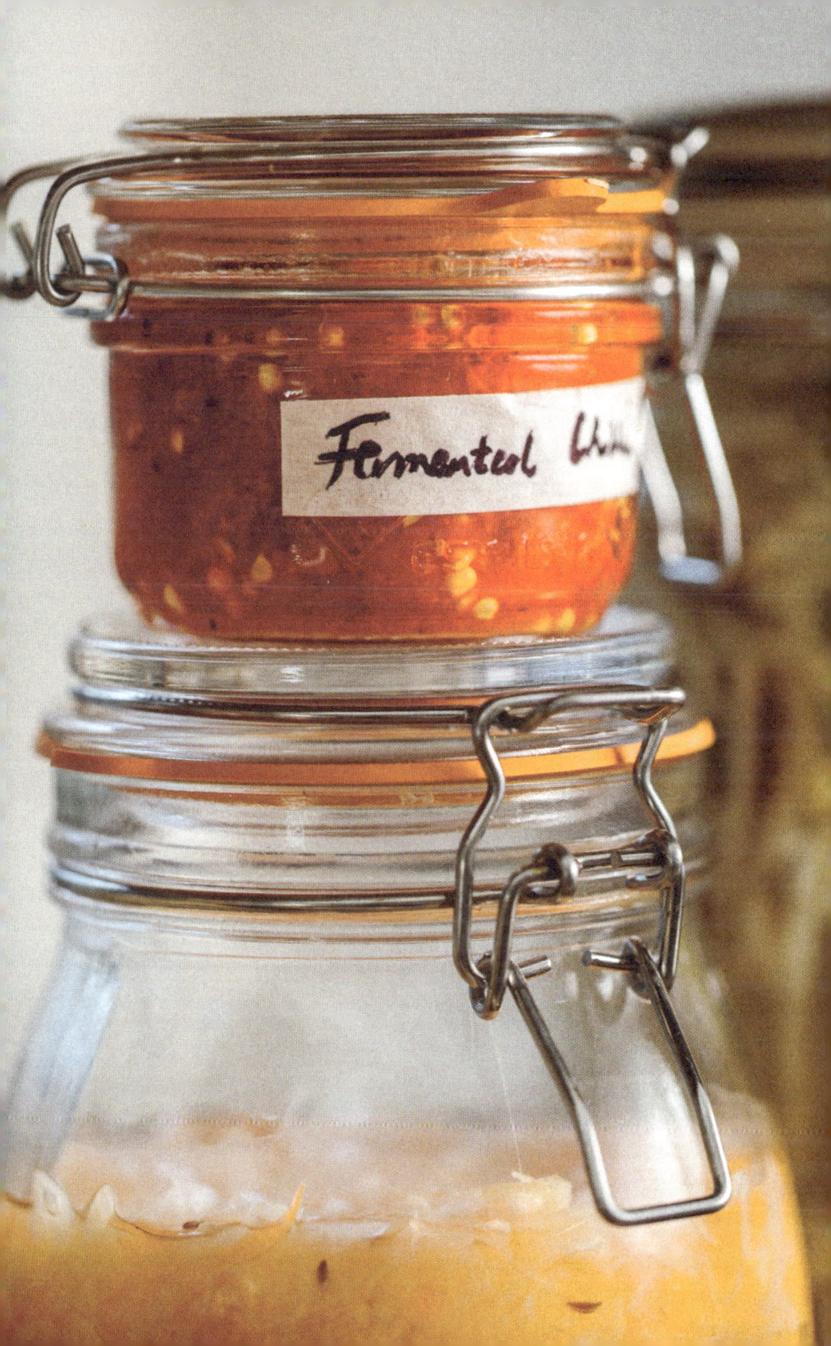
Fermented

Kahm yeast

Kahm yeast is a thin, white film that forms on the surface of fermenting foods due to wild yeast. While harmless to most, it is best to prevent and avoid its development because it increases histamines in the finished ferments. Those sensitive to histamine and wild yeasts should take care here. If you are histamine intolerant and kahm yeast appears on your ferment, consider discarding it and starting over.

Kahm yeast occurs most often when fermenting the Cucurbitaceae family, known as gourds: courgettes, cucumbers, melons, pumpkins, squash and watermelons all fall into this category. Other non-related vine-like plants like grapevines, tomatoes and peppers also see similar yeasts.

Simply add a cling film layer to any ferment to create a barrier inhibiting kahm yeast growth. This layer keeps the ferment anaerobic, which yeasts cannot survive. If kahm yeast arrives at any point during fermentation, wipe it away with a clean cloth and re-cover your ferment with cling film.

Storage

Once fermentation has visibly stopped, everything is free of kahm yeast and tastes superb, you can transfer your ferments from their fermenting vessel into a freshly cleaned and washed jam jar or clip-top vessel and store them in the fridge. Ziplock bags also work well; vacuum-sealed pouches are the pinnacle of preservation as they remove all air. Label them with the date the ferment began and the date it went in the fridge — 'future' you will thank you!

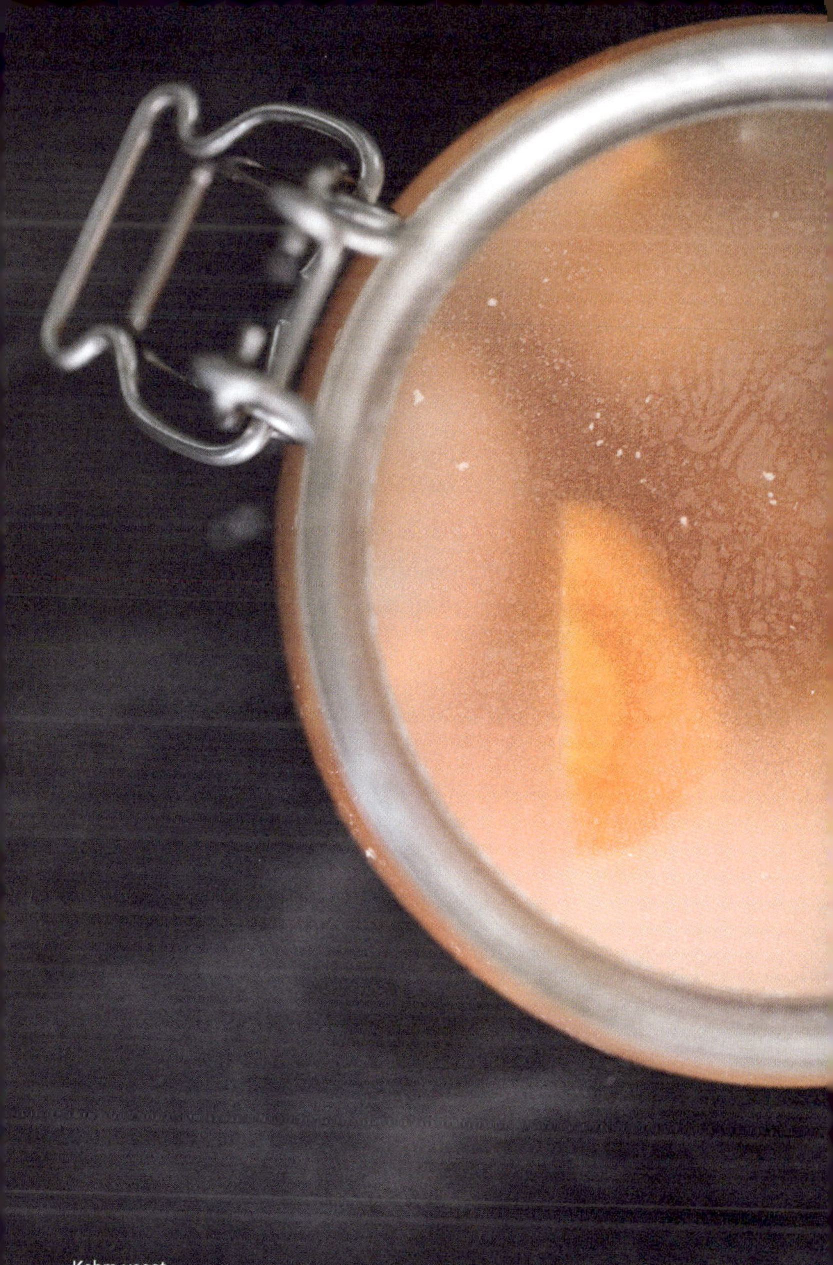

Kahm yeast

Ferments can be kept for many months in the fridge; as long as they remain below pH 4.5. If you plan on keeping a ferment for longer than a month, investing in a pH meter is recommended. Here are a few other things to note:

— Keep your ferment submerged as you take from the jar. Push the veg down flat to keep it compact and moist.

— Keep the inner walls of your ferment vessel clean by wiping with a clean, damp cloth.

— Gas pressure can build up even at cold temperatures. Occasionally 'burp' your jars, opening the lid for a moment, once a week. They might hiss gently.

— To store ferments long-term in the fridge, make sure the temperature is less than 6°C (43°F).

— Add a neat layer of cling film directly on the surface of the ferment and sprinkle a pinch of salt on top, ensuring a long life of continued microbial development.

After three or four weeks of fermenting, most microbial activity has slowed but not stopped. Remember that microbial succession we discussed earlier? The cooler temperatures of a fridge allow the ferment to continue but at a much slower rate. As long as the acidity is high enough (less than pH 4.5), a ferment can survive at a cool temperature for an undetermined time. pH testing with a pH meter is essential to refrigerate lacto-fermented fruit and vegetables for longer than a month from the refrigeration point.

If you have followed our fermentation method accurately, fermenting for the time instructed in each recipe at 10–18°C (50–64°F), and your ferment has a pH of below 4.5 with no kahm yeast, it is possible to store fermented foods out of the fridge. Try to keep the ferment below 15°C and always test for pH prior to eating. Remember that fermentation of food pre-dates the invention of the fridge, but cool, ambient temperatures aid preservation.

Eating your aged ferments

When you've decided that you want to eat an aged ferment (one month or older), take note of the following:

— Remove from the fridge. Check that all looks visibly fine. No moulds? Good.

— There may be some discolouring at the top of the batch, which is not unusual, but test as described below for certainty.

— Submerge the pH meter into the ferment's liquid. Make a note of this number. You are looking for a pH of below 4.5.

— If it is above 4.5, it will not smell inviting and something has gone awry. Be safe and don't take risks. Discard and start making your next batch.

— If it is below 4.5, you are good to taste and see how the flavour has developed at these cooler temperatures. Enjoy your success!

We've created a flow chart for checking your ferments, see overleaf. This is a useful troubleshooting guide if you suspect there may be issues with your creation.

A troubleshooting guide

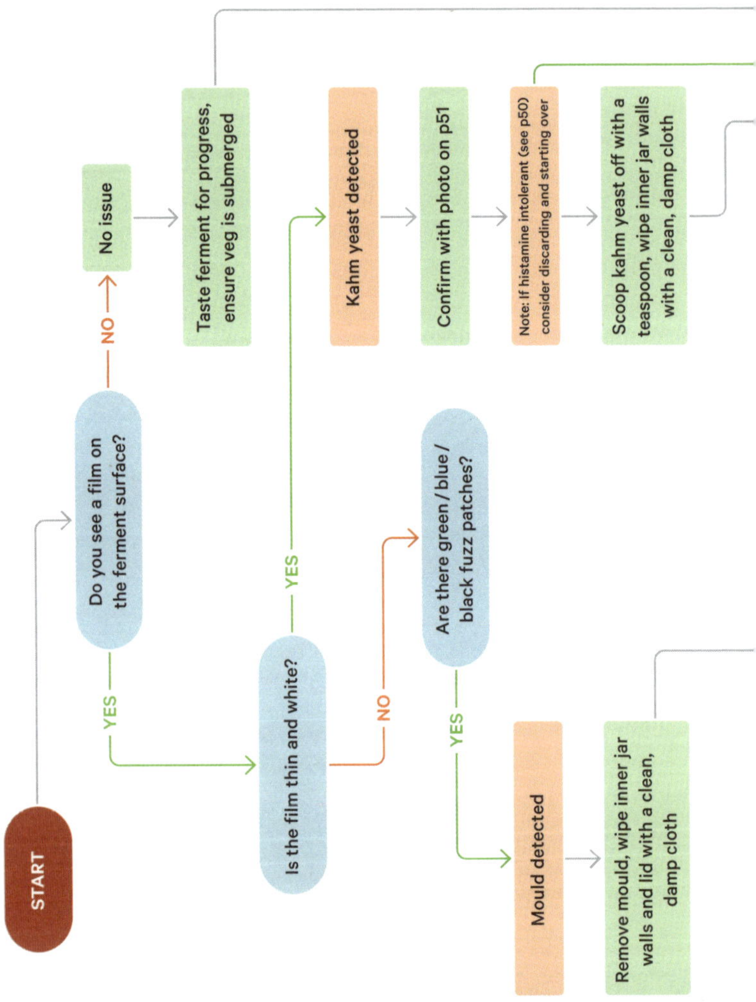

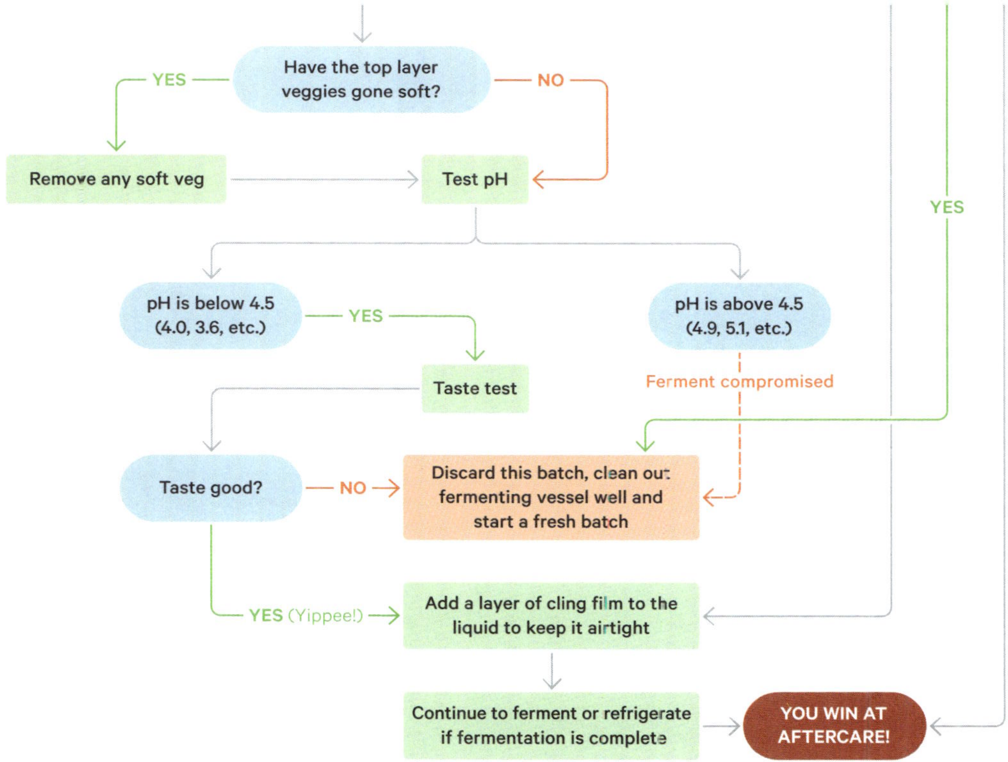
Have the top layer veggies gone soft?
YES
NO
Remove any soft veg
Test pH
YES
pH is below 4.5 (4.0, 3.6, etc.)
pH is above 4.5 (4.9, 5.1, etc.)
YES
Taste test
Ferment compromised
Taste good?
NO
Discard this batch, clean out fermenting vessel well and start a fresh batch
YES (Yippee!)
Add a layer of cling film to the liquid to keep it airtight
Continue to ferment or refrigerate if fermentation is complete
YOU WIN AT AFTERCARE!

How to get the best start from this book

Once you have read the introduction and paid special attention to this before and aftercare chapter, you are ready to get started! Begin with the following recipes:

— Simple or single spiced sauerkraut (page 59/63)
— Tandoor spiced crudiments (page 80)
— Fermented baby carrots (page 79)
— Blackberry and cinnamon shrub (page 130)

After this, start branching out into other ferments. The chart opposite shows how long each ferment usually takes, making it easy to see which could fit into your schedule. At home, we aim to have three food ferments running per month, plus two drink ferments, in an amount that'll see us through while having subsequent batches on rotation ready for the following month. For instance, we usually make on average:

— 1.5kg (3lb 5oz) of sauerkraut per month
— 2 × 1kg (2lb 4oz) jars of brine ferment per month
— 1.7 litres (7 cups) water kefir / kvass / wild soda per week
— 200ml (generous ¾ cup) milk kefir per day

This sees us through each month, although it varies if we are busy or have a little more time on our hands. You may like to be spontaneous, reacting to what's in season or looks good at the greengrocer. You might work best with a plan and schedule, making ferment batches on a specific day of the week. What works for you will be different for someone else. There are no rules! The important thing is to start creating.

Time	Recipes
1–2 days	Milk kefir
3 days	Water kefir
3–5 days	Tepache, Fermented pearl barley
1 week	Shrubs, Bread kvass, Beetroot kvass
1–2 weeks	Peackles, Pine needle soda
10–14 days	Snozzcumbers
3–4 weeks	Sauerkrauts, Fermented wild garlic, Tandoor spiced crudiments, Mushroom condiment, Fermented tomato ketchup and tomato water, Smreka, 'Passionfruit' squash, Fermented baby carrots, Curtido
4+ weeks	Chilli sauce and fermented chilli drops, Lime-fermented shallots, Fermented lime 'pickle', Kimchi
2 weeks–1 year	Mugolio

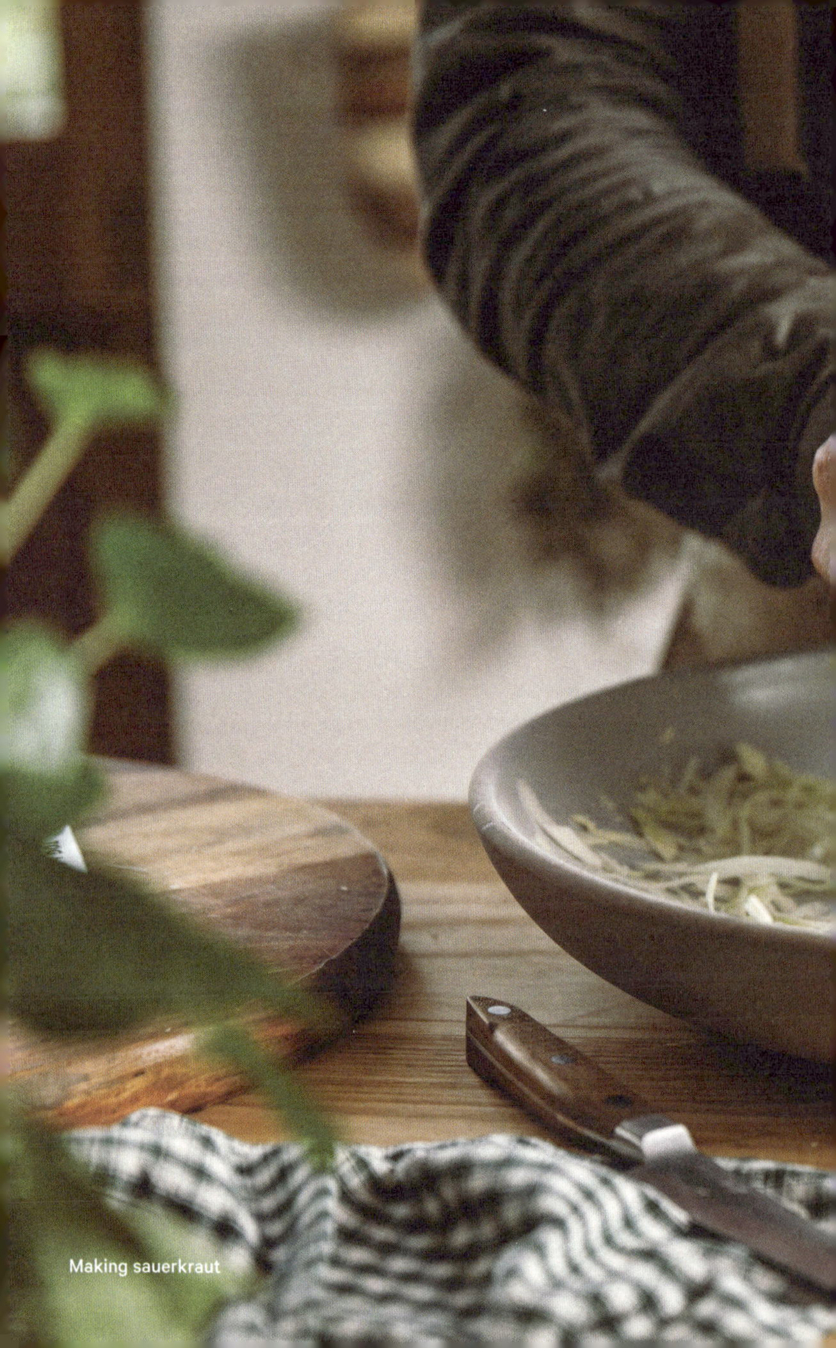

Making sauerkraut

3

Sauerkrauts and other self-brining ferments

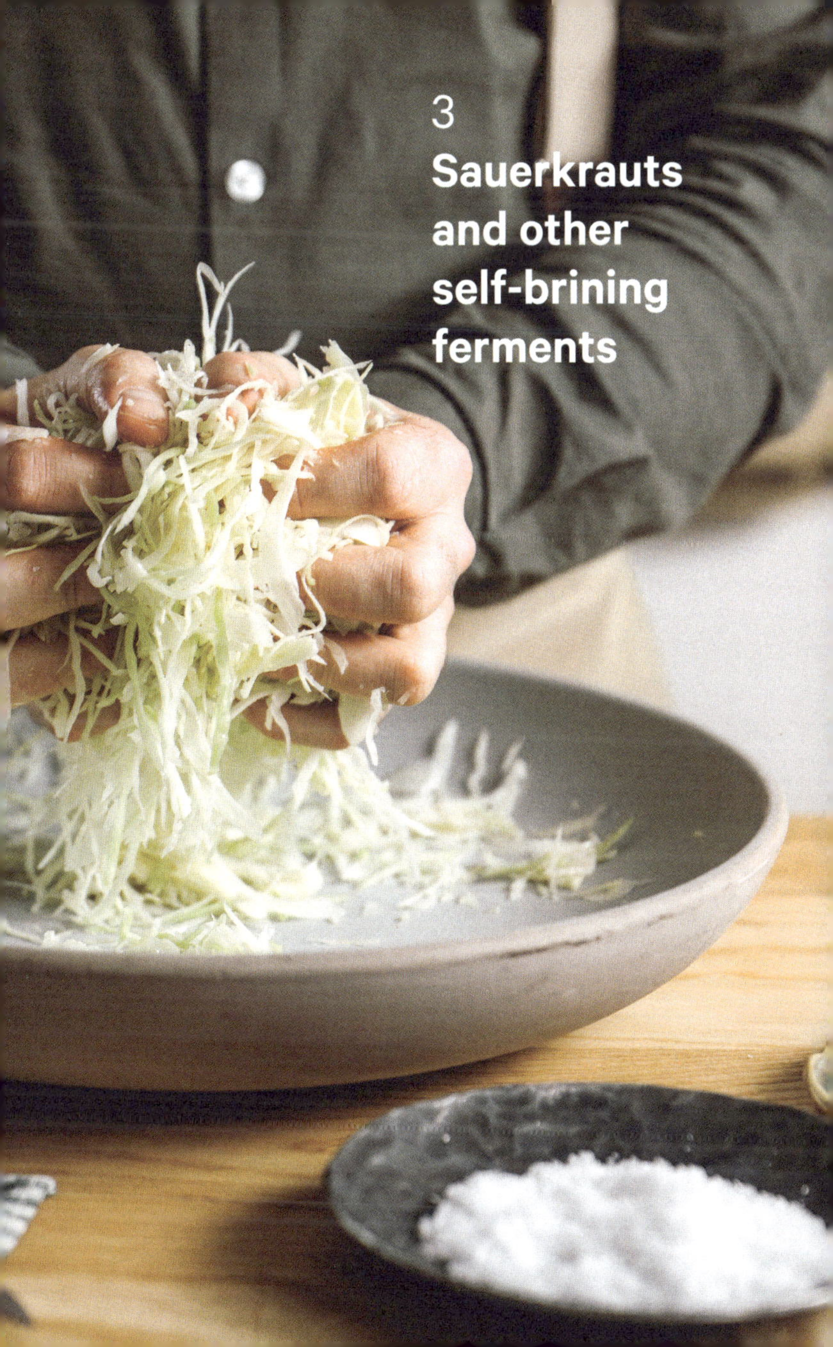

We're naming this section according to a family of ferments that use massaging to create their own brine. No other liquid is introduced, nor should it need to be. You'll coax it out by salting, massaging and wringing, particularly finely sliced vegetables.

Sauerkraut

Certain foods are exquisite because of their simplicity, and sauerkraut is a perfect example. With only two ingredients —cabbage and salt—it is wild that the transformation with microbes creates something so stunning! And it's the perfect starting point to understand successful food fermentation. Following the steps in this recipe, with attention to fine slicing, careful salting and keeping an eye on the temperature for three weeks, you're guaranteed to be hooked on this wonderfully creative process.

The first time you attempt sauerkraut it is worth going for the simple version, to appreciate how much of a transformation our 'microbe farming' makes. For your second batch, bring in a spice of your preference and witness how seductively flavours transform through fermentation.

Simple sauerkraut

KIT: *Clip-top jar or a pair of tessellating tubs. The weight of your cabbage will determine what size vessel you'll need, e.g. 1kg (2lb 4oz) cabbage will require at least a 1 litre (34fl oz) container*

—

white cabbage
natural sea salt

Attention! If you have picked up this book and headed here first, may we urge you to absorb Chapter 2, Before and aftercare to guarantee your sauerkraut success.

First, decide if your white cabbage is dense and fresh or a little older and slightly thirsty. Sometimes, because of cabbages' perceived sturdiness, they may have sat around a while in the food supply chain and benefit from a refresh. Slice through the stem to expose a fresh layer. It may look dry; it may look moist. Generally, the cabbage will feel dense and heavy if it is moist, ideally what we are after.

If feeling a little dry, set the whole cabbage in a bowl in a few centimetres of cold water for a couple of hours to bring life back. It will drink some water, which will help when we compress and squeeze its juices after slicing.

Sauerkraut is best when sliced as finely as possible. Once fermented and with more surface area, the fine slices are better on the tongue; they taste juicier and crisper and carry more flavour and acidity. The ultimate way to achieve thin slices is to use a mandoline set to 'fine'. However, a Y-shaped potato peeler can get cabbage strips very close to this. Slicing with a peeler is more straightforward than cutting with only a knife.

Carefully quarter the cabbage with the stem holding each section together. Next, place a bowl on the scales and set it to zero. Work on the cabbage with the peeler and shred it down as much as possible into the bowl.

Slice the remaining pieces thinly into strips with a knife as best you can. Scoop any escaped cabbage into the bowl as well. Make note of your cabbage weight at this stage. Compost any particularly woody parts of the stem.

Calculate the salt quantity according to the ideal ratio of close to 2%. See pages 29–32.

Shake your salt through the sliced cabbage. Within moments, the salt will act on the surface of the cuts. Moisture is being pulled from the cell walls, which makes our brine.

Now roll up your sleeves and set about squishing that cabbage, see image pages 56-57. It'll take a surprising amount of force so really massage and knead it. You can put the weight of your torso into leaning and squashing it. After about 5 minutes, you'll see that 'the brine from within' flows free when pressing a clump of cabbage together in your hands. There will appear to be less cabbage than there was at the start but much more liquid. You can't really overdo this step. You'll no doubt feel better for taking out your stress on this substantial and stoic cabbage, now melting in your hands. At some point, when you are satisfied, stop.

To test if you have made enough brine, first rescue the sliced cabbage you've gotten all over the countertop and add it to the bowl (waste not, want not). Level the cabbage flat and see if it will submerge in its brine with a gentle, constant push with the palm of your hand. If so, we have enough brine to create an air-free environment in our

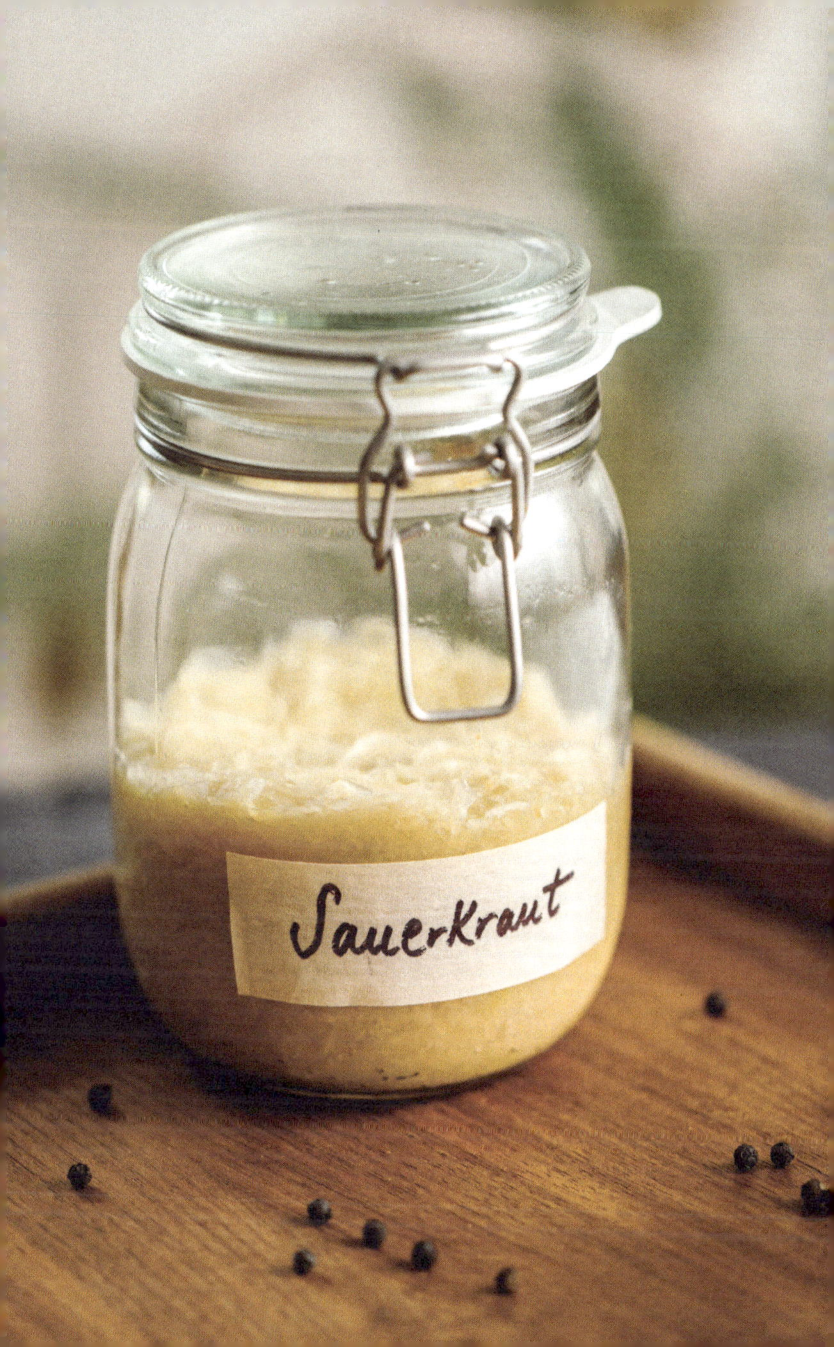
Sauerkraut

fermenting vessel. More liquid will be pulled from the cabbage over the coming hours through the osmotic action of the salt on the vegetable cell walls and we shouldn't need to add any more water.

Important step: It is essential to taste at every opportunity. You'll get a mustardy whoosh from all those sulphur compounds being worked upon by enzymes. An alchemical 'cooking' is happening right under your nose. When you taste you might find the 2% salt level a bit much, not unpleasantly, but saltier than one would ordinarily season food. That saltiness will diffuse over time. The salt is currently concentrated on the surface of the cabbage and has yet to work into the cells. Later on, acidity increases from forming lactic acids, counteracting the salt taste. In fact, in the finished ferment, it'll be barely perceivable.

Pack your cabbage into your chosen vessel. If using tessellating tubs, push the cabbage as flat as possible and wipe down the sides of the tub with a clean, wet cloth. Add a layer of cling film, then your second tub and weigh down with a lidded jam jar with water inside. If you are using a glass fermenting jar, fill your jar, leaving headspace of 2.5 cm (1 in) for the arrival of bubbles. If you have ferment weights, add them; if not, use a layer of cling film to cover the surface of the cabbage.

Place your ferments in a tray to catch any leaks. In the coming days, check the temperature, watch for bubbles and ensure your soon-to-be sauerkraut is happily submerged. Refer back to page 41 to follow your ferment's progress over the next 3–4 weeks and don't forget to taste the developing sauerkraut as you tend to its needs.

Spiced sauerkrauts

Now that you have made your first batch of sauerkraut, we encourage you, for your second sauerkraut batch, to experiment with adding a single spice. Add 1 teaspoon per kilo of cabbage of one of the following tried-and-tested favourites: allspice, aniseed, celery seed, cardamom, caraway, coriander seed, cumin, fennel, juniper, mace, mustard seed, nigella seed, nutmeg, peppercorn, sumac.

Sauerkraut can be a canvas for so many flavour experiments. Epic spice blends in sauerkraut include: black garlic and dulse (seaweed), cumin and dried apricot, nutmeg and saffron, coriander seed and orange zest.

In essence, sauerkraut is fermented cabbage but the lesser-starchy roots (carrots, beetroot, celeriac, daikon, parsnip, jicama, Jerusalem artichokes and swede) make happy additions to a cabbage ferment. Sometimes, they are a little low in moisture to create enough brine from within, so keeping two-thirds of the weight as cabbage is a good solution. If you have a veg box, this can be a great way to use more of it. Read on for other recipe ideas.

A note on radishes and turnips

How should we put this? When we've fermented these in their pure form, the results have always been far too stinky for our olfactory systems. One time, on a catering job in a cute country cottage, we had to jettison fermented radish into a far field because of the honk. They can be used though. You can include 5 per cent in a kimchi recipe, but we've found these strong mustard roots too funky when fermented beyond this. Call us what you will; there's undoubtedly somewhere in the world where this phenomenon is celebrated, just not here.

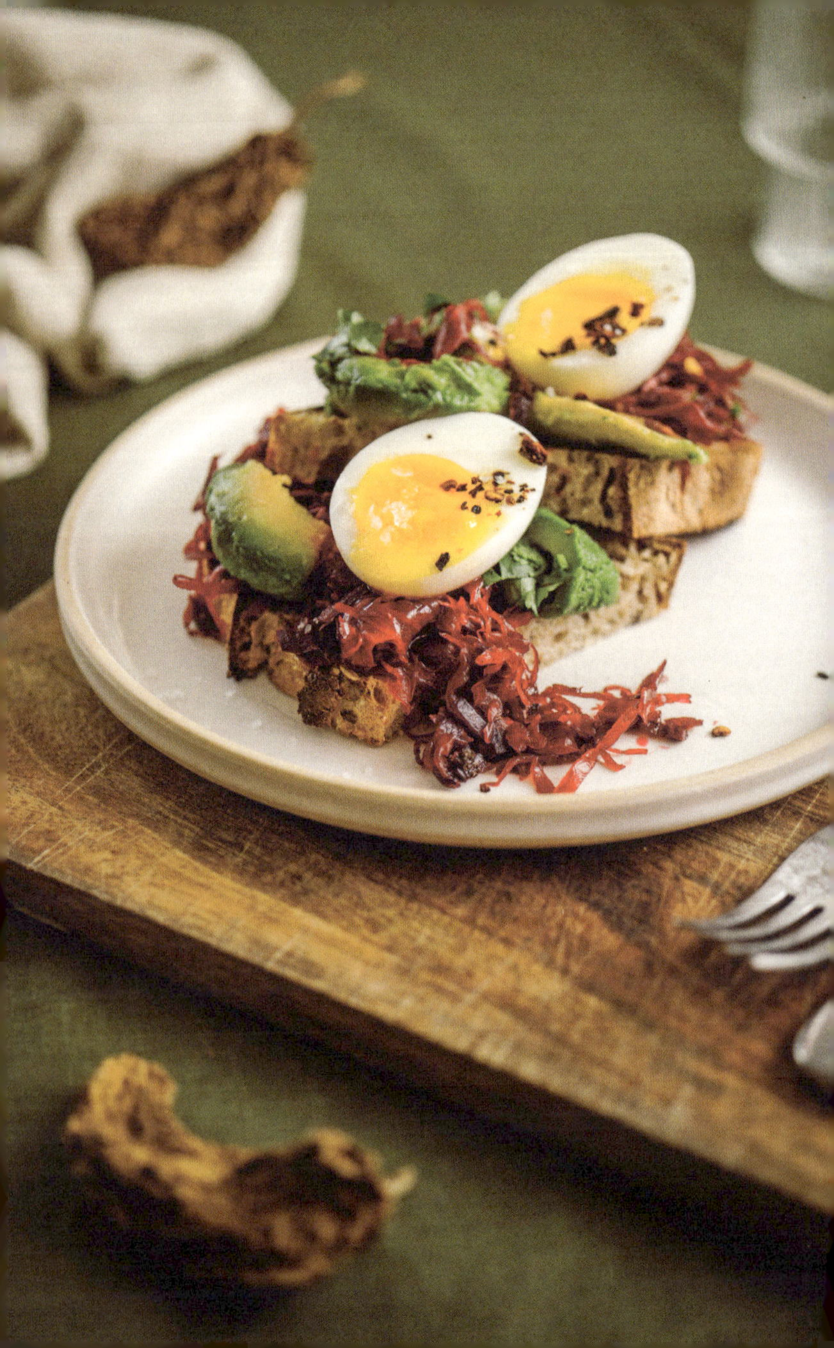

Beetroot and caraway sauerkraut

Beetroot has some excellent sweet and earthy notes, which lend well to fermentation. We have fermented it as the sole ingredient in beetkraut, which tastes delicious, but on every occasion, the texture is gelatinous and thick. Great for a Halloween theme, but perhaps not for everyone? When used as a third of a sauerkraut recipe, it imbues bright colour and that great taste without thickening proceedings too much. Caraway is a happy partner in this recipe; its pepper and aniseed tones, delicate bitterness and earthiness ties this sauerkraut together with joy.

KIT: *Clip-top jar or a pair of tessellating tubs*

—

70% white and/or red cabbage
30% raw beetroot, grated
1 tsp caraway seeds per 1kg (2lb 4oz) veg
natural sea salt

Follow the method for simple sauerkraut on page 59. After the squeezing stage, mix in the caraway and grated beetroot before leaving it to ferment in your chosen vessel.

SERVE WITH: *Any dish where the egg yolk is intact — that yellow and purple is a feast for the eyes. Avocado brings a pleasant fattiness to this ferment, so roughly chop half an avocado, fold it into the kraut, spread over sourdough toast, top with a poached egg and dust with chipotle flakes and fresh coriander. Marvellous. This kraut also goes well with smoked or cured fish.*

Ginger, carrot and turmeric sauerkraut

To avoid having permanently yellow paws from raw turmeric, massage the cabbage, carrot and salt in the same way as plain sauerkraut. When complete, stir in the sliced turmeric with a spoon before packing it into your ferment vessels.

KIT: *Clip-top jar or a pair of tessellating tubs*

—

70% white or red cabbage
30% carrot, finely grated
a large thumb of fresh ginger, grated
a thumb of fresh turmeric root, washed well and finely sliced
natural sea salt

Follow the method for simple sauerkraut on page 59, adding the turmeric at the final stage.

SERVE WITH: *This makes a great pairing with Asian dishes. Add a spoonful to top noodles, curries and ramen.*

Jicama, jalapeño and lime sauerkraut

Jicama is a Mexican root with many qualities. It is juicy, crisp and has a sweet flavour. It's high in fibre and rich in inulin, a prebiotic that feeds gut flora deep within the bowels — a winner on all fronts. This extra-juicy sauerkraut is made using equal parts of the two main ingredients, with lime zest and green jalapeño chilli bringing brightness.

KIT: *Clip-top jar or a pair of tessellating tubs*

—

50% white cabbage
50% jicama root, peeled
zest of 1 lime per 1kg (2lb 4oz)
2–6 green jalapeño chillies, to taste (or use dried chipotle flakes for a smoked alternative)
natural sea salt

Follow the method for simple sauerkraut on page 59, but to avoid spicy hands, put the chillies in after you've squeezed the cabbage to bring out its moisture. Then, pack into your fermenting set-up in the usual manner.

This ferment is the least likely to make it to the recommended 3 weeks of fermenting without getting raided. It's just so good.

SERVE WITH: *Bring the ferment to room temperature, then pour warm, rendered bacon fat through it. The moment you try this, you'll realise how good a ferment can be when paired with a fatty lipid. This works with any meat roasting drippings. If meat is not your thing, use lightly warmed avocado or olive oil instead. Serve as a slaw with pan-toasted pure corn quesadillas with Oaxaca cheese, feta or cottage cheese, scattered with coriander leaves. You'll be in a happy place.*

Swedekraut

We've flipped a buttery swede and carrot mash that usually appears only at Christmas lunch into a ferment—hurrah! Swede is underutilised as a vegetable, even though it appears much more often across the year and it's ace in a ferment. Its silky sweetness cries out for the mellow part of the nutmeg plant, mace blades. Adding mace might make you feel a little nostalgic with its homely, autumnal, earthy, chopped wood scent. This unusual sauerkraut is otherworldly when served with the warm toffee notes of caramelised brown butter—see the recipe below. You'll never forget it.

KIT: *Clip-top jar or a pair of tessellating tubs, tall-sided saucepan, shallow baking tray that fits inside your sink*

—

50% white cabbage
40% swede, peeled and finely grated
10% carrot, finely grated
3–4 mace blades per 1kg (2lb 4oz) of veg
natural sea salt at 2% of total weight

For the brown butter

250g (9oz) salted butter

Follow the method for simple sauerkraut on page 59, making sure you shred your cabbage as thin as angel hair and the swede and carrots are finely grated. The finer the grate, the more buttery the resulting recipe becomes.

When you are ready to serve, make the brown butter. Caramelising butter solids is simple, but express care needs to be taken: 1, not to over-caramelise the butter, and 2, not to splash the molten butter on yourself as you prepare it. (Clarified ghee makes a good substitute; just warm it lightly before adding to the slaw you are serving.) Don't start this recipe until:

- You have 15 minutes free from any distractions.
- You have a clear sink with a shallow baking tray inside, topped with water — to quench your hot saucepan.
- Your kitchen is calm and free from people and bustle.
- You've read this recipe twice.

With a tablespoon in hand, a tea towel over your shoulder or an oven mitt to hand, melt the butter in a small, tall-sided pan over a medium heat. Continue to cook; after a few minutes, you'll see white milk solids break loose, down under the oil layer. Keep a close eye on it as after a few more minutes, the whole pan will foam up. Carefully stir the foaming butter and tilt the pan. Under the foam, the milk solids will stick and catch to the pan and start to brown — they can go from brown to black relatively fast. The butter fat itself will start to look lightly caramel. When a nutty aroma hits the air, turn off the heat.

Now, with a tea towel between you and the handle of the pan, slowly lower the pan into the tray of water in the sink and watch out for steam and spitting. Despite the quench, the pan will be very hot for some time.

Transfer the pan back to the safety of a rear hob and allow to cool for about 20 minutes. Then, leaving the burnt solids in the pan, slowly pour the caramel butter fat into another container and discard the burnt milk solids. There will be less than 210g (7oz) of burnt butter due to water evaporation and milk solid loss.

Add melted brown butter to swedekraut that has been gently warmed without fully cooking it (the kraut is alive and probiotic up to 37°C / 98°F). Store any leftover brown butter in the fridge. Brown butter is very stable and will last more than a month in the fridge.

SERVE WITH: *This is delicious with any meal where mashed potato happens. Pair it alongside freshly grilled white fish and capers. Dish up anywhere you know it will bring joy.*

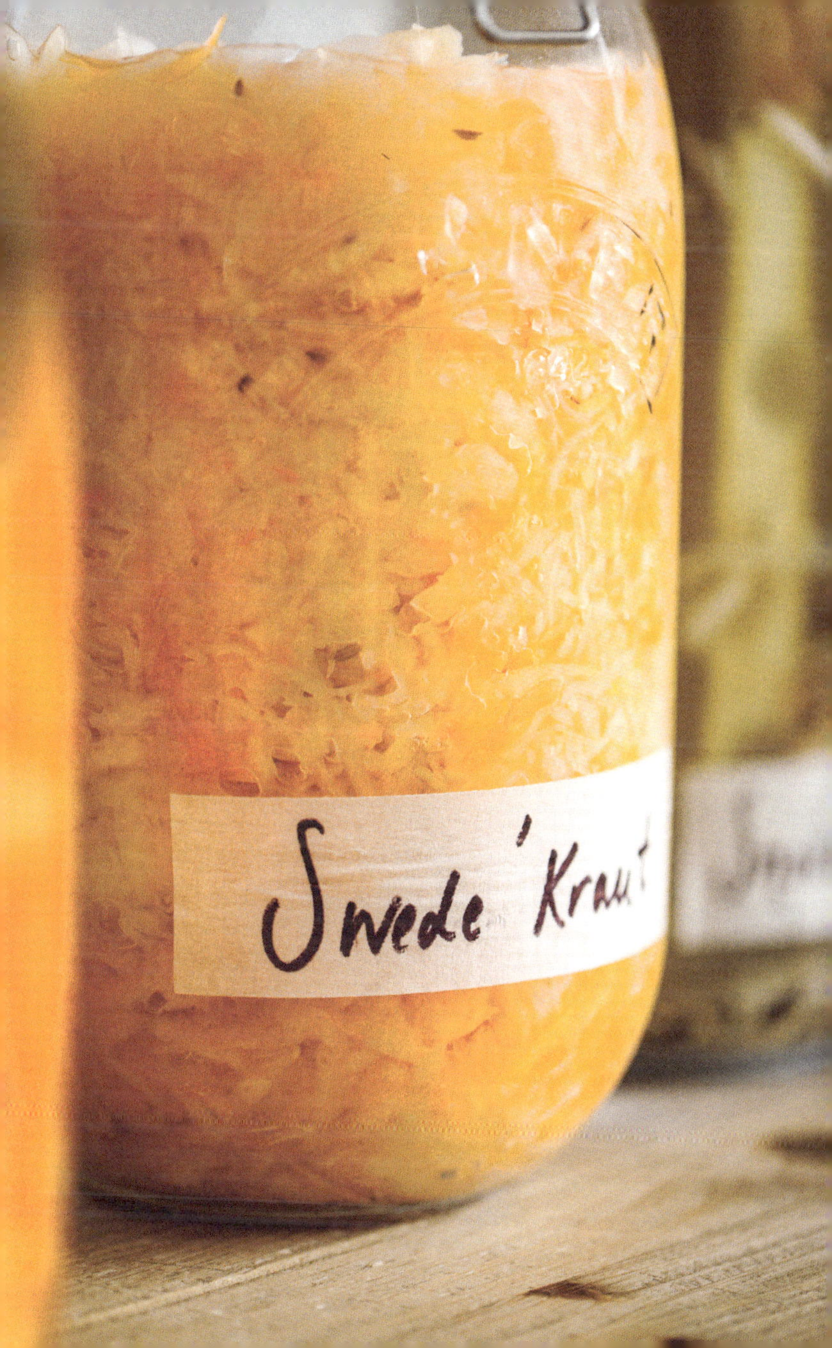
Swede 'Kraut

Curtido

Originating from Salvador but popular across Central America, this fermented slaw is vibrant and intriguing. Its main herb, Mexican oregano, is a trove of fascinating tastes. It's often found as a dried herb, and if you enjoy Italian oregano's warmth, you'll undoubtedly love it. It has a neat hit of aniseed, is less menthol and more lemon zest-like.

Slaws like curtido and coleslaw suit fermentation superbly, and until the modern-day use of fridges, we suspect that they would have traditionally been ferments in their own right rather than side salads. Be free in your ratios; see these fermented slaws as an opportunity to use what you have, even if the ratio differs from what we describe below.

KIT: *Clip-top jar or a pair of tessellating tubs*

—

50% white and/or red cabbage
25% carrot, finely grated
25% onion / spring onion / red onion, finely sliced
2–6 green jalapeño chillies per 1kg (2lb 4oz) of veg, to taste
zest and juice of 1 lime per 1kg (2lb 4oz) of veg
1 tsp dried Mexican oregano per 1kg (2lb 4oz) of veg
natural sea salt at 2% of total weight

Follow the method for simple sauerkraut on page 59. You'll be adding chilli peppers and don't want spicy fingers, so stir these in after you've squished and massaged the other ingredients together.

SERVE WITH: *Curtido would traditionally be served with corn pupusa flatbreads, refried beans and melted cheese. This bright and floral ferment suits a wide variety of foods. You can use it as a slaw on a whole gamut of dishes and salads.*

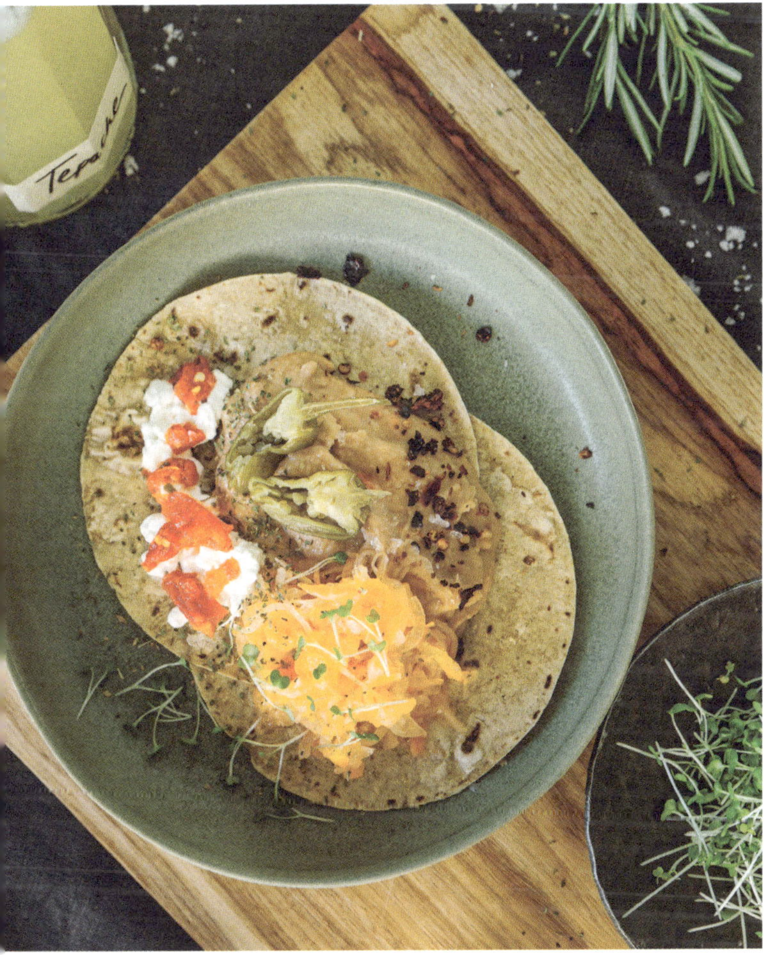

Fermented wild garlic

This two-part recipe is a great way to ensure you can preserve wild garlic for the whole year and make pesto on demand. A winning recipe to make with kids, it involves an adventure to gather your wild garlic leaves first.

Consult a foraging guidebook (see Resources) so that you are sure that you are picking the correct plant. Wild garlic grows in woodland, forests and riversides from late winter to late spring and it helps that wild garlic smells... garlicky! Pick responsibly—just a handful here and there—and only pick the leaves as the bulbs take seven years to mature.

KIT: *Clip-top jar*

2 big bunches of wild garlic leaves
natural sea salt

First wash your leaves in a salad spinner or a clean sink full of cold water and shake thoroughly, then chop them into 1 cm (½ in) strips, including the stems. Set a large bowl on your scales and set to zero, add the wild garlic leaves and calculate 2% of the weight. Add this amount of sea salt, sprinkling it through the leaves to disperse.

As with cabbage in sauerkraut, the wild garlic will start to give off water; when combined with the salt this creates a brine, which will ferment the leaves. Massage, knead and squeeze the leaves until you have enough liquid to cover it all when pushed down. You'll probably need to add a splash or two of water here to make enough brine.

Press your leaves into your jar, covering them with the brine and ensuring everything is under the liquid. Add a layer of cling film to the surface of the ferment.

Leave to ferment at room temperature for 3–4 weeks. It will start to bubble after a few days, indicating fermentation has begun. Release the lid every now and then to let off some gas. After roughly one month, the bubbling will stop, and your ferment is ready for the fridge.

SERVE WITH: *The delicate chive-like scent will take you back to the day you foraged this and brightens omelettes, salads, roasted vegetable dishes, rice and noodles.*

Fermented wild garlic pesto

If you like, follow the recipe below to turn your fermented wild garlic into a delicious pesto.

KIT: *Food blender / processor, jar to store finished pesto*

—

150g (5oz) fermented wild garlic, strained of brine
150ml (⅔ cup) olive oil
50g (2oz) grated Parmesan
zest and juice of 1 lemon
150g (5oz) nuts (pine nuts, cashews, walnuts, hazelnuts all work well; use a mixture if that's what you have)
natural sea salt, to taste (optional)

Add all your ingredients except the salt to a blender or food processor. Blend until it reaches your desired consistency. Taste and add salt if needed. Pour into a clean jar and store in the fridge for up to 1 week.

SERVE WITH: *Stir into soups, into stews, use as a pasta sauce, brighten pizzas and elevate a sandwich toastie filling.*

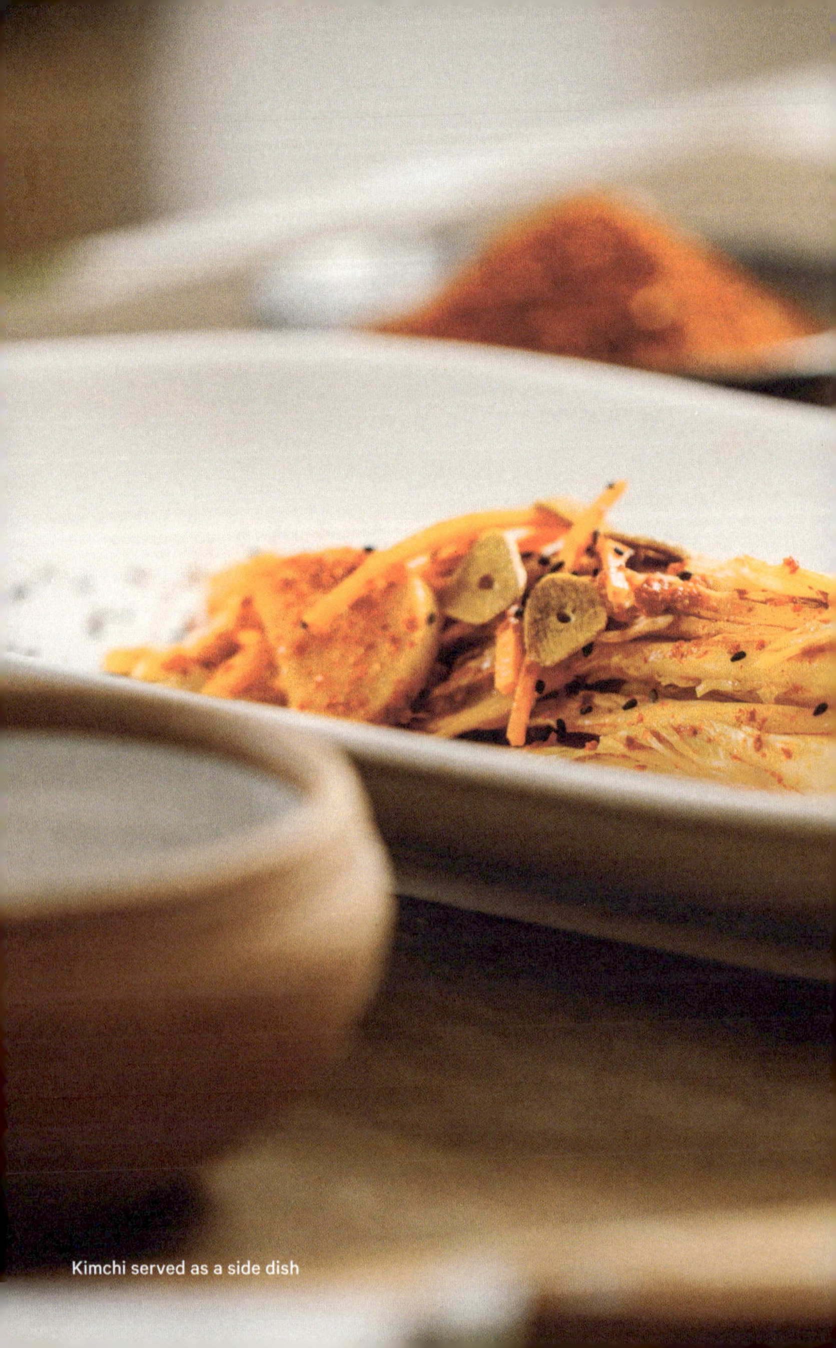

Kimchi served as a side dish

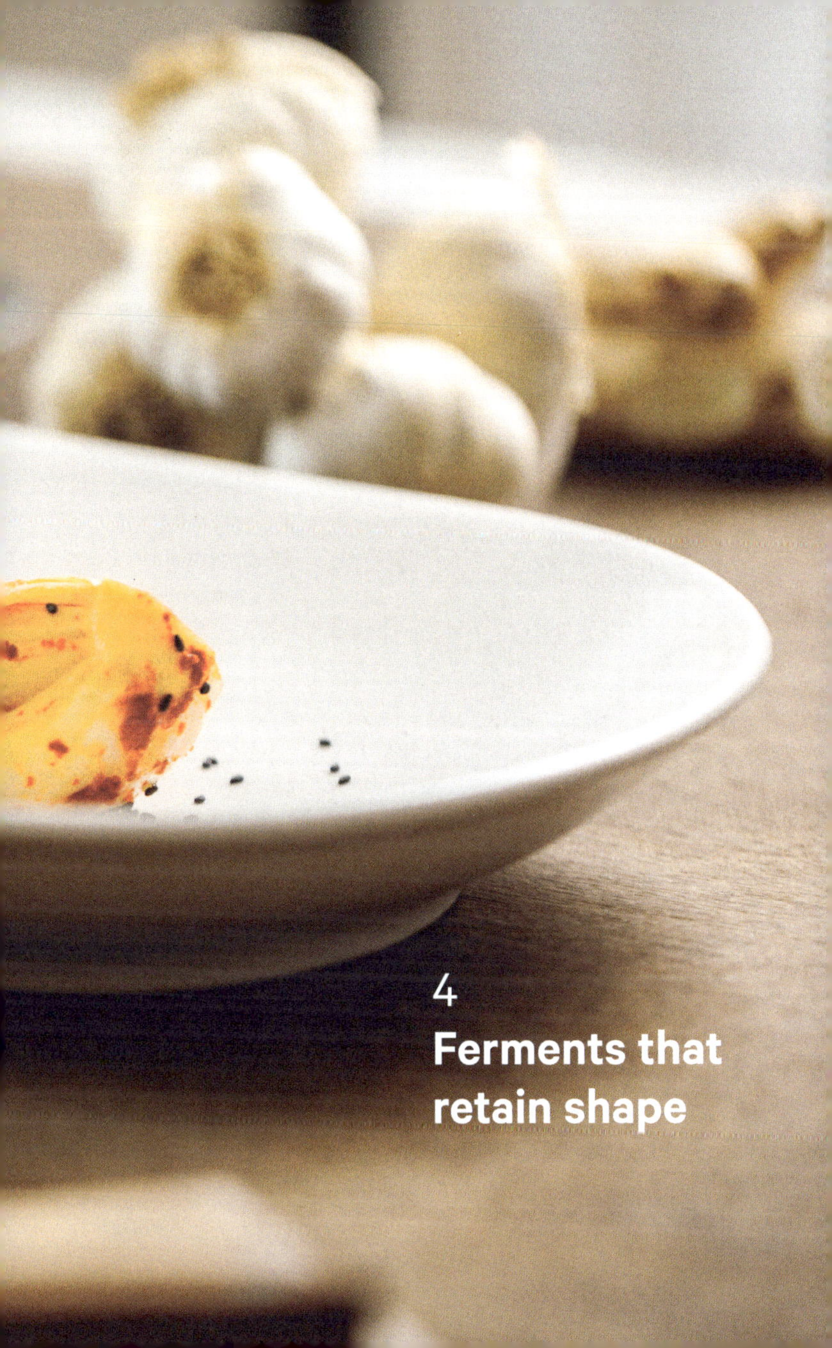

4

Ferments that retain shape

There are many times in vegetable fermentation where finely slicing vegetables and shredding them to obscurity is a missed potential. Some have beautiful forms. Think how a romanesco cauliflower has wild interlocking spirals in its florets, representing how plants grow in Fibonacci patterns (see page 25). Fresh garden peas have an undeniable form, with their joyous little pops of green. Mushed up, not so cheerful. So, let us ferment those beautiful shapes whole in a way that celebrates nature.

Brining is the process of adding salt to liquid and then immersing vegetables. Over time the salt will evenly disperse, seep into the vegetable cells, pull liquid from within, crisp things up and bring vegetable essence to the brine.

As in life, too much salt is a bad thing, but too little, and it'll go rogue. Remember that the salt quantities are easy to calculate; just like the sauerkrauts we'll be following the same 2 per cent salt rule (see pages 29–32). There is one main exception here, the snozzcumbers, which prefer a ratio of 2.5 per cent.

We can ferment all sorts of vegetables and fruits in brine in all sizes of vessels—limitless possibilities await. As always, if you have picked up this book and headed here first, may we urge you to absorb Chapter 2 to guarantee success.

Fermented baby carrots

If you want something easy to start with, try this simple and delicious ferment. Warming spices such as coriander seed, cumin, star anise and fennel seed also work well.

KIT: *Clip-top jar*

—

carrots (Chantenay or baby carrots work well)
a few sprigs of thyme
2 crushed cardamon pods per 500g (1lb 2oz) of veg
water
natural sea salt

Scrub the carrots to remove any soil residue. You can leave the skins on or peel them if you prefer. Small carrots can be left whole, and larger carrots chopped up so that all pieces are equal in size — roughly that of your thumb.

Place your jar on the scales and set to zero, then fill the jar with carrots, herbs and spices, and top up with water until everything is submerged. Take note of the total weight, then calculate 2% of this in salt. Add the salt to the jar, clip the lid on and leave on the kitchen work surface out of direct sunlight.

After a few days, you should notice bubbles forming, indicating fermentation has begun. Leave for at least 3 weeks for maximum flavour. Once fermentation is complete, store in the fridge at 5°C (40°F).

SERVE WITH: *Delicious as crudités for lunch, picnics, or pre-dinner nibbles. Sneak them into your children's lunchbox to dip in houmous or cream cheese.*

Tandoor spiced crudiments

Before beginning a main meal, having some raw food is wise. They have had this spot-on in France for eons, eating crudités before dinner. Embracing fresh batons of raw garden produce alleviates hunger, primes digestion and awakens our 'gut pet' (or microbiome) for what is next to come.

Building on the idea of raw, with its slow microbial 'cooking', we introduce our beloved tandoor spiced fermented crudités or 'crudiments'. This is a recipe that marks our introduction to fermentation some two decades back, a recipe that, at the time, we had no idea was a ferment.

An old scribbled-down, copied, photocopied-again, cauliflower pickle recipe was circulating. We suspect it must have originated from a Madhur Jaffrey cookbook. Something was intriguing about this recipe, which is probably why it was doing the rounds among the food-obsessed, and a couple of close friends dared to attempt it. It wasn't long before we tried it, too.

Apart from loads of really bold spices and aromatics, the one part of the recipe that felt challenging was when it instructed to leave the mixture out on the worktop to fizz and bubble for a week or more—everything our food-hygiene-trained selves had learned not to do! This recipe did not mention fermentation; no one talked about lactobacillus back then. It called for 15g (1 tablespoon) of salt for a 500g (1lb 2oz) jar, which at roughly 3% is a bit high on reflection.

After a week of fizzing, we needed to pull on our brave boots and taste the cauliflower chunks, but what a revelation! They were saline and hot, hot, hot from the chilli, ginger and garlic but at the same time mellowed and ever-so moreish. Incredible.

Despite an in-depth search, we have failed to find the original recipe. However, we know this to be a ferment and we have been able to play around with the concept, and so can you! A batch is never the same twice because of all the ingredients you can substitute for what you have to hand, but it is worth starting each time with a cauliflower and a few carrots. This recipe allows us to be root-to-shoot frugal, using the entirety of the cauliflower, leaves, stems and all. You'll end up with 1–2kg (2½–4½lb) of ferment.

KIT: *Clip-top jar or a pair of tessellating tubs*

—

1 cauliflower, ideally organic
5 carrots
1 bulb of garlic
a 'pinky' of fresh turmeric root
a big thumb of fresh ginger
2–10 fresh green or red chilli peppers, halved lengthways, seeds in place
1 heaped tbsp tandoor masala curry blend
1 heaped tbsp ground turmeric
1 tsp nigella seeds
1 tsp a spice you love
water
natural sea salt

Get hands-on with the cauliflower. If you have kids, get them involved in breaking the florets from the cauliflower stalk. Let them explore the shapes within and play. Interactions like this are vital to developing a child's healthy relationship with food. Roughly cut the stalk into bite-sized chunks and slice the leaves and stems. Make fanciful carrot shapes. Peel the garlic cloves and slice them in two along their length. Garlic is so good fermented. The slow process breaks down the pungent volatile compounds of allium and makes them very edible. The result of fermenting garlic is an enriched superfood that now doesn't repeat on a burp.

Wash the turmeric root well, but don't peel it as it will stain your hands. Peel the ginger to eliminate any soil residue. (A chef's tip: a teaspoon point will peel ginger superbly.) Slice it and the turmeric however you want it to be in the finished ferment.

Place your jar or container on the scales, set to zero, then load up all the ingredients, cover with water until all ingredients are fully submerged and make a note of the weight. Add 2% of this weight in salt to the jar. Add a layer of cling film to cover the surface and place the jar in a tray to catch any overspill.

SERVE WITH: *As a pre-dinner crudité for curious and adventurous friends.*

This tandoor spiced ferment recipe can be anything you like. We've enjoyed it with the hotter vindaloo spice blend and had fun crossing continents and making a Caribbean jerk spiced or Japanese furikake variant. The possibilities are as adventurous as your spice cupboard and can help you use up spices bought for a recipe you only cooked once. Stay curious.

The cure for boredom is curiosity.
There is no cure for curiosity.
Dorothy Parker

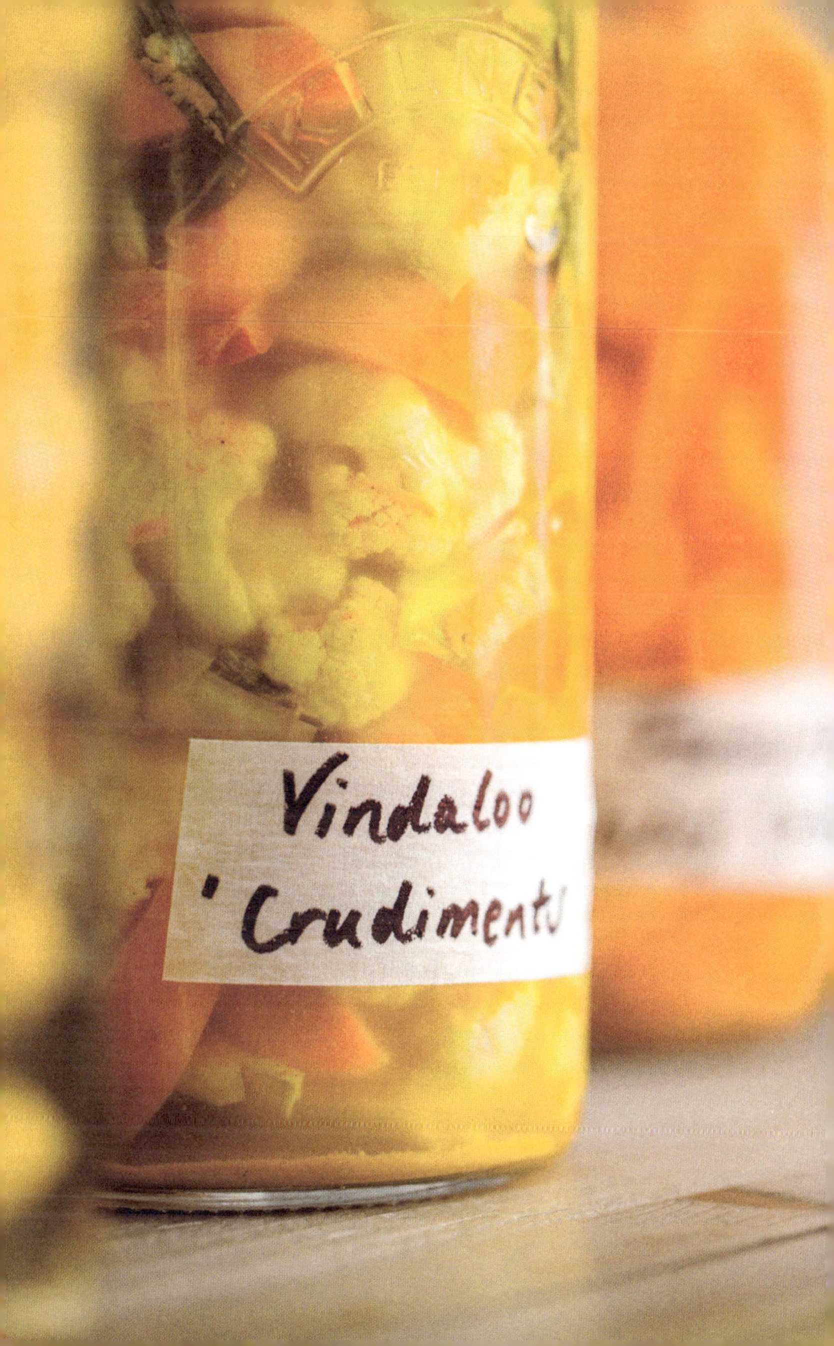
Vindaloo
'Crudiments'

Peackles

Peackles are, by far, one of our favourite ferments and the one with the cutest name, conjuring up a jar of little smiling peas! The results are zingy little pops of summer and a fun ferment for kids.

KIT: *Clip-top jar*

—

peas (frozen can be used; just defrost them first)
a few mint or lovage leaves (optional)
water
natural sea salt

Place your empty jar on the scales and set to zero. Add the peas to the jar, plus any herbs, and top up with water until all peas are submerged, leaving about an inch of headroom at the top of the jar. Take note of the total weight, then calculate 2% of this in salt and add to the jar. Give it a little mix, then clip the lid on. Leave on the kitchen work surface out of direct sunlight. See image on page 148.

After a few days, you should notice bubbles indicating that fermentation has begun. We recommend leaving them for 3 weeks for maximum flavour. However, we understand it may be difficult to wait this long! Your fermented peas will be ready from 7–12 days. Ensure all peas are fully submerged and no kahm yeast has formed. (Follow the steps in Chapter 2: Before and aftercare to prevent kahm yeast growth.) Once ready, store in the fridge at 5°C (40°F).

SERVE WITH: *These are the perfect topping for pasta dishes, risottos or sprinkled in salads. A favourite lunch of ours is toasted sourdough with cottage cheese and rocket leaves, sprinkled with peackles.*

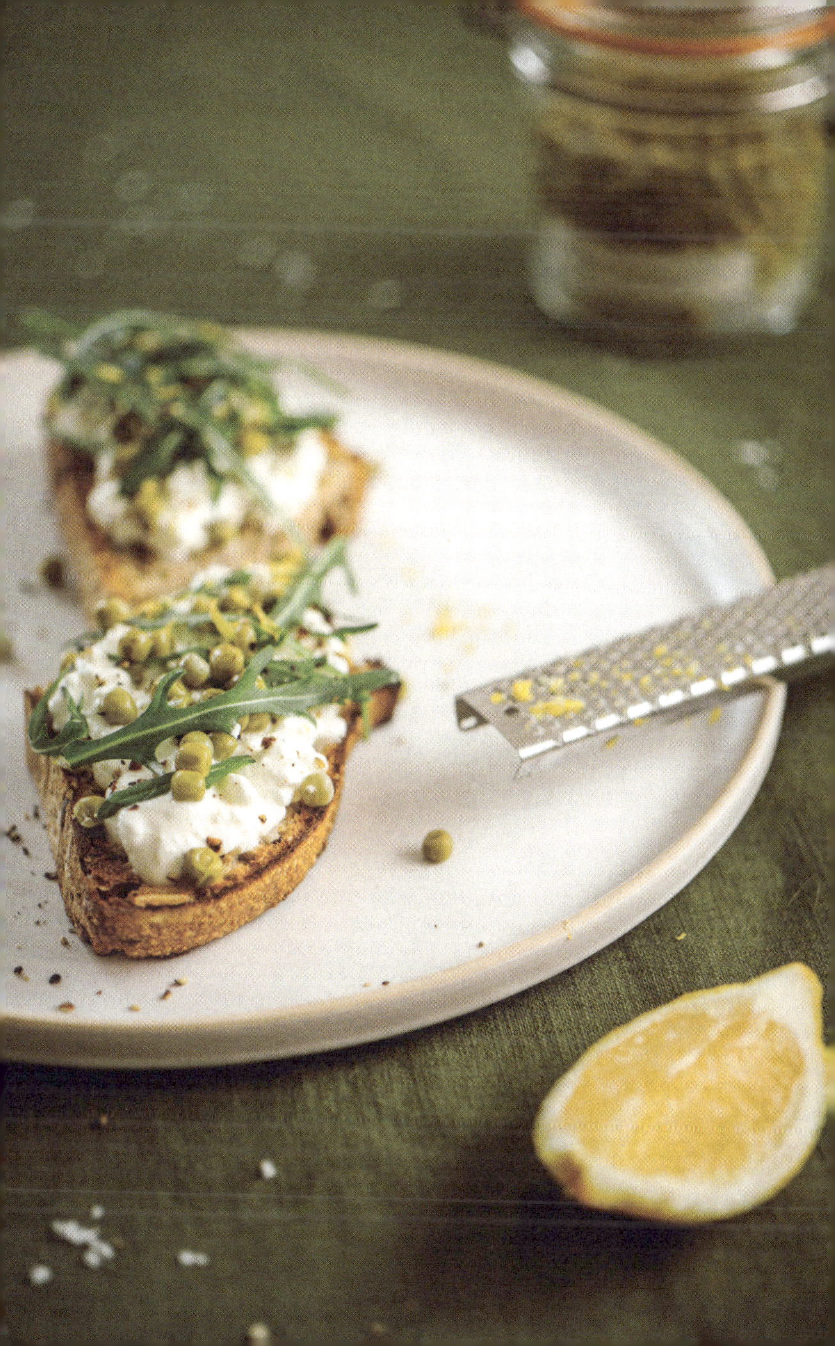

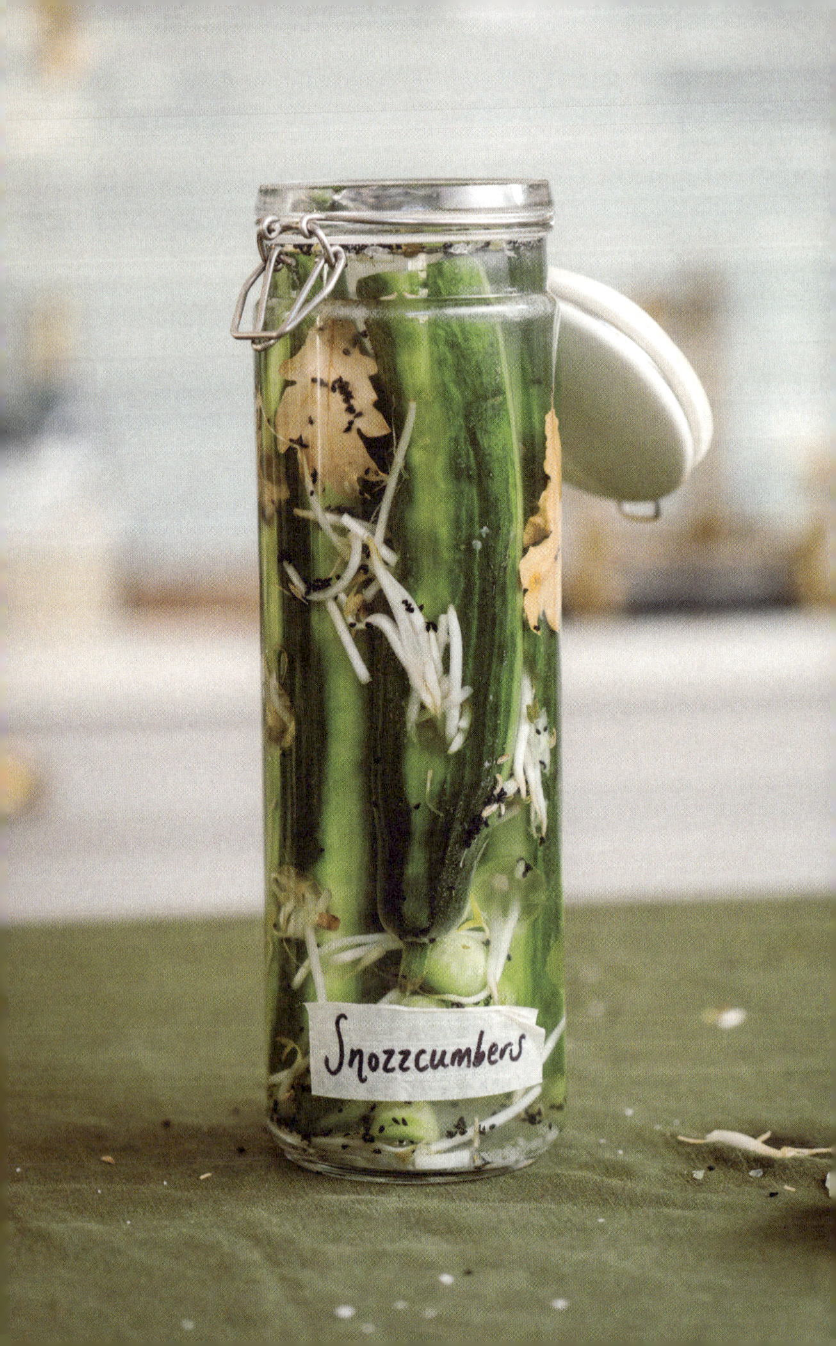
Snozzcumbers

Snozzcumbers

> **It was a long, striped, knobbly thing, a bit like a cucumber, but black and white instead of green.**
> Roald Dahl, *The BFG*

This is such a fun recipe to make with children! It gets them playing and interacting with the ingredients, tasting the bits you aren't using and creating a visual triumph inspired by Roald Dahl's *The BFG*.

You can use mini cucumbers or larger ones chopped up. We added beansprouts and nigella seeds to get the full effect, but you can also leave those out to make a simple cucumber ferment.

KIT: *Tall clip-top jar*

—

2 cucumbers
150g (5½oz) beansprouts, as fresh as you can find
nigella and mustard seeds, about 1 tsp total spices per 1 litre (4 cups) of ferment
4 oak leaves (see page 34)
natural sea salt
calcium chloride (optional — see page 34)

First prepare the cucumber. Peel alternate strips of the skin so that you have a striped effect and trim off the ends. Using a long butter knife or similar, remove the soft, seedy part in the middle in a 'corkscrew' action. If you find this difficult, chop each cucumber in half to make it easier to reach down the middle. Gouge out a few holes in each cucumber for visual effect.

(recipe continues page 90)

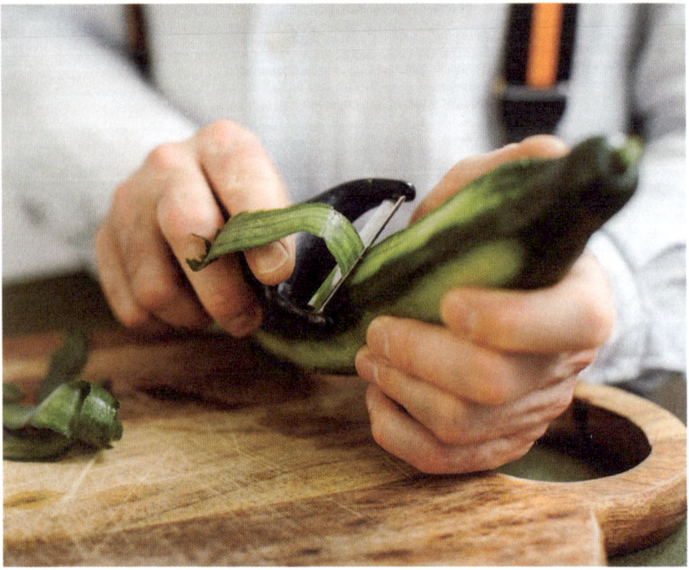

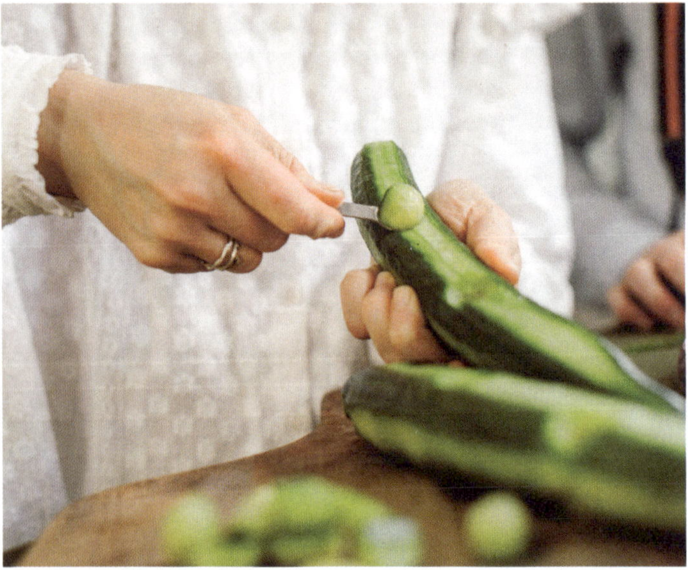

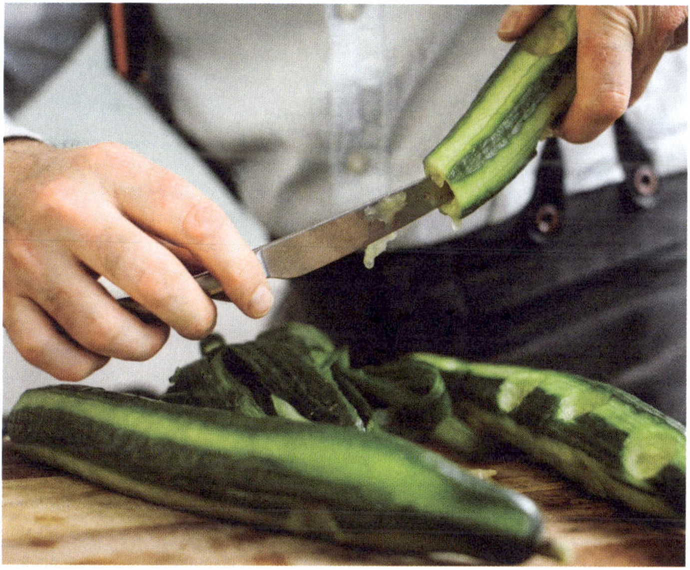

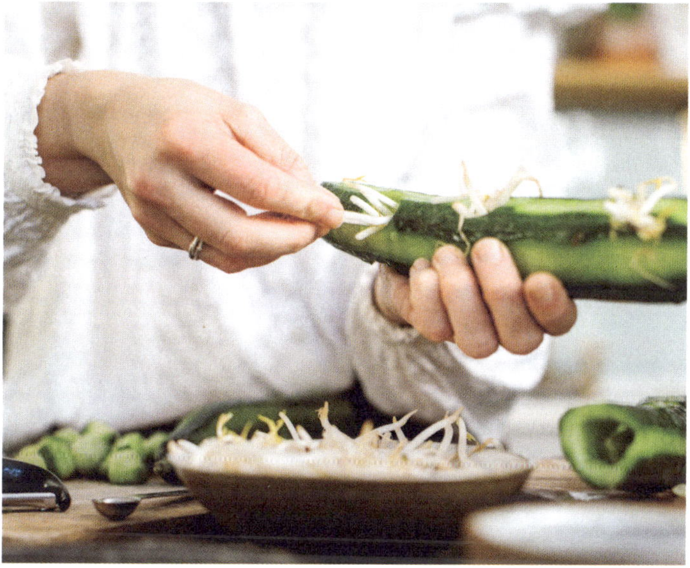

Snozzcumber preparation

Stuff the hollows with beansprouts. Pack in as many as possible, leaving the rest loose in your ferment jar.

Place your tallest clip-top jar onto your scales and set it to zero. Stand the cucumbers upright in the jar and sprinkle them with the remaining beansprouts, nigella and mustard seeds and oak leaves. Top with cold water, filling the jar until everything is covered. Make a note of the total weight.

Calculate the salt needed at 2.5%. Cucumbers tend to soften during fermentation so they need a little more salt than in our other recipes. For 1kg (2lb 4oz) total weight, you need 25g (around 4 tsp) salt. If you have no natural tannin-rich leaves to hand, add a touch of food-grade calcium chloride to help keep the cucumbers crisp (for every 1kg (2lb 4oz), add 1g (1/5 tsp) calcium chloride).

Add the salt and calcium chloride, if using, and ensure everything is below the brine's surface. A layer of cling film resting on the surface can protect it from any kahm yeast formation. Clip on your lid and leave it at room temperature. Your fermented snozzcumbers will likely be ready between 10 and 14 days, depending on the temperature of your room.

SERVE WITH: *These fermented snozzcumbers make a great party piece. Equally, they're a fun topping or side dish to a mac and cheese, noodle or rice dish or simply as a snack. Dice into smaller pieces to serve as a garnish.*

'Passionfruit' squash

The Flavour Thesaurus by Niki Segnit is a book every flavour gastronaut should have in their library. Niki explores the realms of taste within ingredients and suggests a multitude of complementary ways in which to pair them. Most of all, it encourages you to stop and think about taste, which is a skill as advantageous as it is rewarding and one that is explicitly valuable in fermentation.

Inspired, we started creating thoughtful spice combinations. As that journey progressed, we happened across something that astonished us. On an intuition, we took some cubed squash and added coriander seeds, cinnamon sticks and a sparing amount of cloves before brine-fermenting it. Coriander seeds have a citrus, lemony, floral, Earl Grey tea-like woodiness. Science boffins say that these tropical notes come from the terpene linalool.

We were not ready for what happened by the end of the fermentation, and we urge you to try this yourself. For some crazy reason, once the acidity has peaked and all those compounds have unravelled, the resulting taste is passionfruit. Exactly passionfruit? Make some, and you'll see for yourself.

Squash is a slightly starchy gourd that occasionally turns soft through fermentation. When this happened to us, we went with it, strained the solids and blended them. We now had a passionfruit purée fit for use in puddings! To avoid the softening effect, add 0.1% of calcium chloride to your ferment — no more than 1g (1/5 tsp) per 1kg (2lb 4oz).

(continued overleaf)

KIT: *Clip-top jar*

1 squash (Crown Prince is our favourite, but experiment with other varieties)
2 tsp coriander seeds per 1kg (2lb 4oz)
1 cinnamon / cassia stick per 1kg (2lb 4oz)
2 cloves per 1kg (2lb 4oz)
natural sea salt
calcium chloride (optional, see page 34)

First prepare the squash: peel, deseed and cut the soft flesh into 1–2 cm (½ in) cubes.

Place your jar on the scales and set them to zero, then fill the jar with squash chunks and spices and top up with water until everything is submerged. Take note of the total weight and then calculate 2% of this in salt. Add the salt to the jar, as well as the calcium chloride, if using. Clip the lid on and leave on the kitchen work surface out of direct sunlight.

After a few days, you should notice bubbles forming, indicating fermentation has begun. We recommend leaving these for at least 3 weeks for maximum flavour. After this time, once fermentation is complete, store in the fridge at 5°C (40°F).

SERVE WITH: *The passionfruit flavours here make a perfect pairing to ceviche, white fish, prawns and white crab meat. We love it as a topping in fish tacos!*

Other vegetables we recommend fermenting with herbs and spices:

— **Bell peppers** *pair with basil / oregano / rosemary / thyme*
A lovely fusion, however, similar to squash, tomatoes and cucumbers, fermenting peppers are prone to harbouring kahm yeast on the surface — see page 48 for how to deal with this.

— **Garlic cloves** *pair with rosemary / thyme / parsley / tarragon / basil / paprika / chilli / ginger*
The antioxidants, vitamins and minerals in garlic are even more accessible to the body after fermenting, making this a beneficial, quick and healthy ingredient to have in your larder. Don't throw away the brine once you've eaten all your cloves — it's excellent splashed into hot lemon and honey water to help combat colds and flu. Often, when fermenting garlic, the process can turn the cloves blue or green. There's nothing to worry about — it's just the lactic acid produced during lacto-fermentation reacting with sulphur compounds in the garlic. They're perfectly safe to eat when this happens.

— **Beetroot** *pair with aniseed / cumin / caraway / star anise*
Brine-fermented beetroot is a wonderful fusion of earthy, sweet flavours. Use the brine in salad dressings, in borscht, or add a shot measure to your daily smoothie.

— **Onions** *pair with celery / cloves / garlic / ginger / mint / rosemary / sage*
We love fermented red onions as a topping for dhal, hot dogs, or open sandwiches.

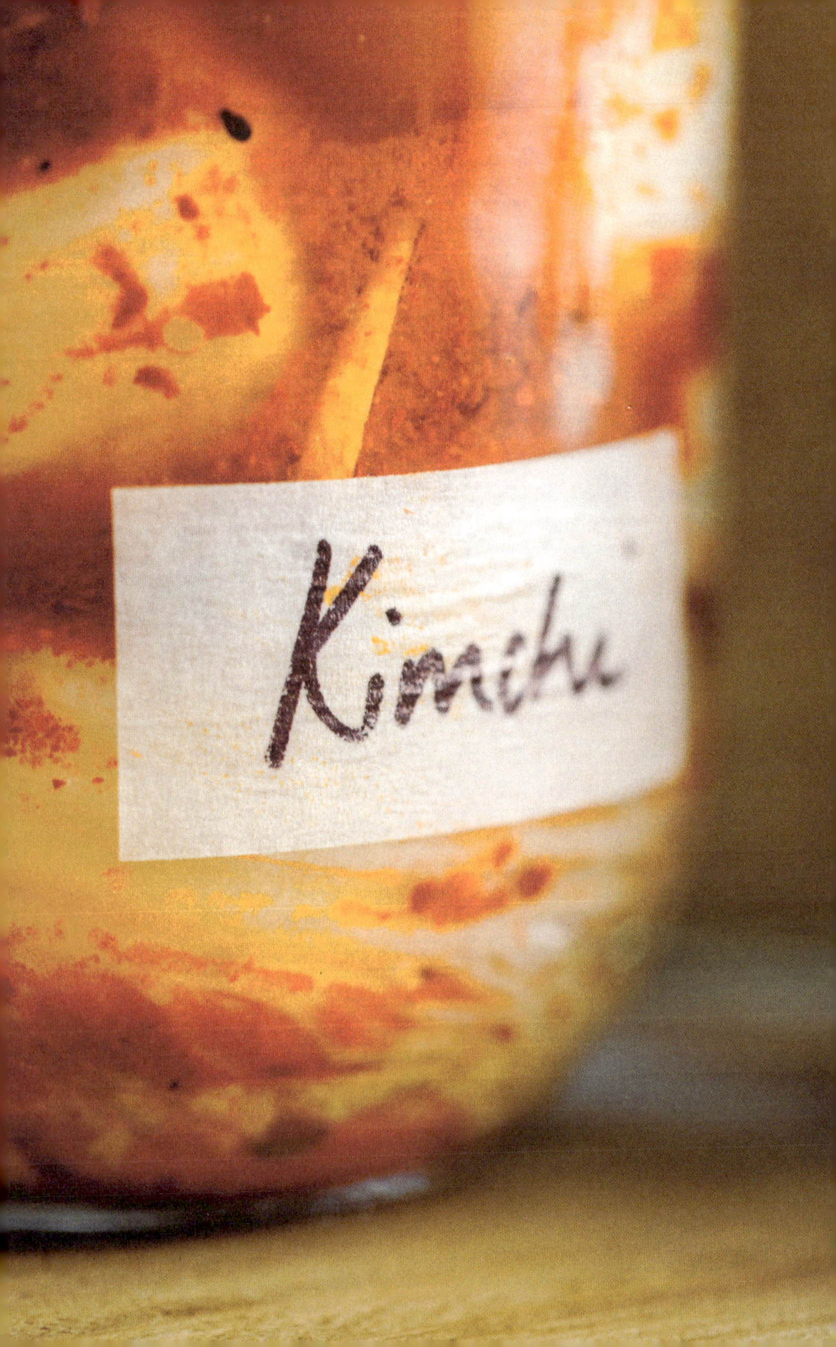
Kimchi

Kimchi

Here is an excellent opportunity to create your family recipe for kimchi, Korea's traditional side dish. Once you have followed the recipe below to make your first batch, you can find your own interpretation and spice blend the next time you make it. When perfected, be proud of your creation and pass it on.

A step that will add a certain prettiness to the finish of this kimchi is to tear open the fresh cabbage into four pieces, the entire length of the cabbage. The large quarter pieces with their torn frilled leaf edges look fantastic as a finished ferment. To achieve this (while looking like British strongman legend Geoff Capes ripping up Yellow Pages phone books), you shall first make two cuts in a cross shape at the base of of the cabbage. This will give you some leverage to pull apart the remainder of the cabbage, first in half, then each half into quarters.

There are two steps in the fermentation process to make your kimchi a success. Chinese (Napa) cabbages contain a lot of liquid so an initial brining is required to shrink the leaves and make them more pliable before they go down for their full ferment with spices and additional vegetables.

We use fish sauce in this recipe, which contains some of the salt we need to ferment here and adds a wonderful umami flavour. If you'd like to keep it vegetarian, just leave it out and adjust the amount of salt added (see method).

KIT: *Pair of tessellating tubs or a clip-top jar large enough to fit all your ingredients, ferment weights*

—

1 Chinese (Napa) cabbage
natural sea salt
4 garlic cloves, finely sliced and fried until golden

a thumb of fresh ginger, peeled and julienned
a thumb of fresh galangal, peeled and julienned
100g (3½oz) daikon radish, peeled and cut into half-moon slices
100g (3½oz) carrot, peeled and julienned
2 tbsp Korean red pepper flakes, plus extra to taste
fish sauce (see below)

Quarter the cabbage through the stem at the bottom and evenly tear it open. Place your jar or tub onto the scales and set it to zero. Add the cabbage and pack it down into the bottom. Pour enough water to completely cover the cabbage and note the total weight. Calculate 2% of this and add this weight in salt. Clip on your lid or tessellate your second tub as a lid. Add a jar filled with water to weigh it down. Leave at room temperature for 48 hours.

After 48 hours, it is time for stage two. Drain the cabbage wedges, keeping the brine liquid aside as you'll need it later.

Mix the garlic, ginger, galangal, radish and carrot in a bowl with the Korean red pepper flakes. Loosen with a little of the brine you saved from the cabbage, then add your cabbage wedges to the mixture. Give everything a good mix to coat the cabbage wedges with the vegetable spice blend.

Pop your jar back on the scales and set it to zero. Pour the kimchi mixture into the jar and make a note of the weight. This time, add 1% (of the 2% required) in sea salt and make up the rest of the salt content using fish sauce.*

---

* The brand of fish sauce we use states on the label that it is 20% salt, which means that 100ml of fish sauce contains 20g of salt. In our example the total mixture weighs 1kg, which means we want 10g of salt using sea salt and 10g of salt from fish sauce, therefore we added 50ml of fish sauce. Make sure you adjust your calculations accordingly.

If you are vegetarian, omit the fish sauce and add 2% salt here instead.

Pack all ingredients into your fermentation vessel, ensuring they are all fully submerged. If you need to, top up the level with the brine you set aside. If you have one, you can weigh down the cabbage mix with a pickle pebble. A layer of cling film works well if you don't.

Clip the lid on your jar, or, using the tessellating tub method, cling film the base of a clean tub and push it inside your tub of ingredients to act as a lid and add a jar filled with water on top (see image on page 39–40).

Ferment at room temperature (10–18°C / 50–64°F) for 4 weeks. Regularly check the temperature and cabbage submersion — anything above the liquid line risks spoiling, so keep it all tucked under the brine.

After about a month, once fermentation is complete, store in the fridge at 5°C (40°F). If you've used tubs, transfer your kimchi (plus brine) to a jar to reuse the tubs for your next ferment. The jar will also take up much less space in your fridge.

Feel free to experiment with spice levels and ingredients once you're comfortable with the recipe. Use dried seaweed and shiitake mushrooms to make the brine; there are many ways to play and riff on our recipe.

SERVE WITH: *Enjoy kimchi in a myriad of ways. It is just incredible in a cheese toastie or on grilled cheese, as a side to ramen, noodle or rice dishes and with eggs, especially omelettes.*

Fermented pearl barley

Fermenting pearl barley grains before cooking brings an incredibly rich, creamy, umami flavour to dishes, as well as helping them to retain an excellent bite. We don't need salt here — the barley's natural starch content provides sufficient food for microbes to thrive, leading to fermentation.

KIT: *Tub or container with lid*

—

pearl barley
water

Pour your pearl barley into a tub and cover with cold water. If you live in an area where tap water is treated, it's best to use filtered water or water that has been boiled and left to cool. Ensure the grains are completely covered and pop the lid on. Leave on the kitchen work surface out of direct sunlight. After 3–5 days, drain the grains, rinse in fresh water and cook as usual.

SERVE WITH: *Fermented pearl barley adds an incredible depth to risottos, stews, soups and salads. One of our favourites is a fermented pearl barley broth with chicken and heaps of vegetables.*

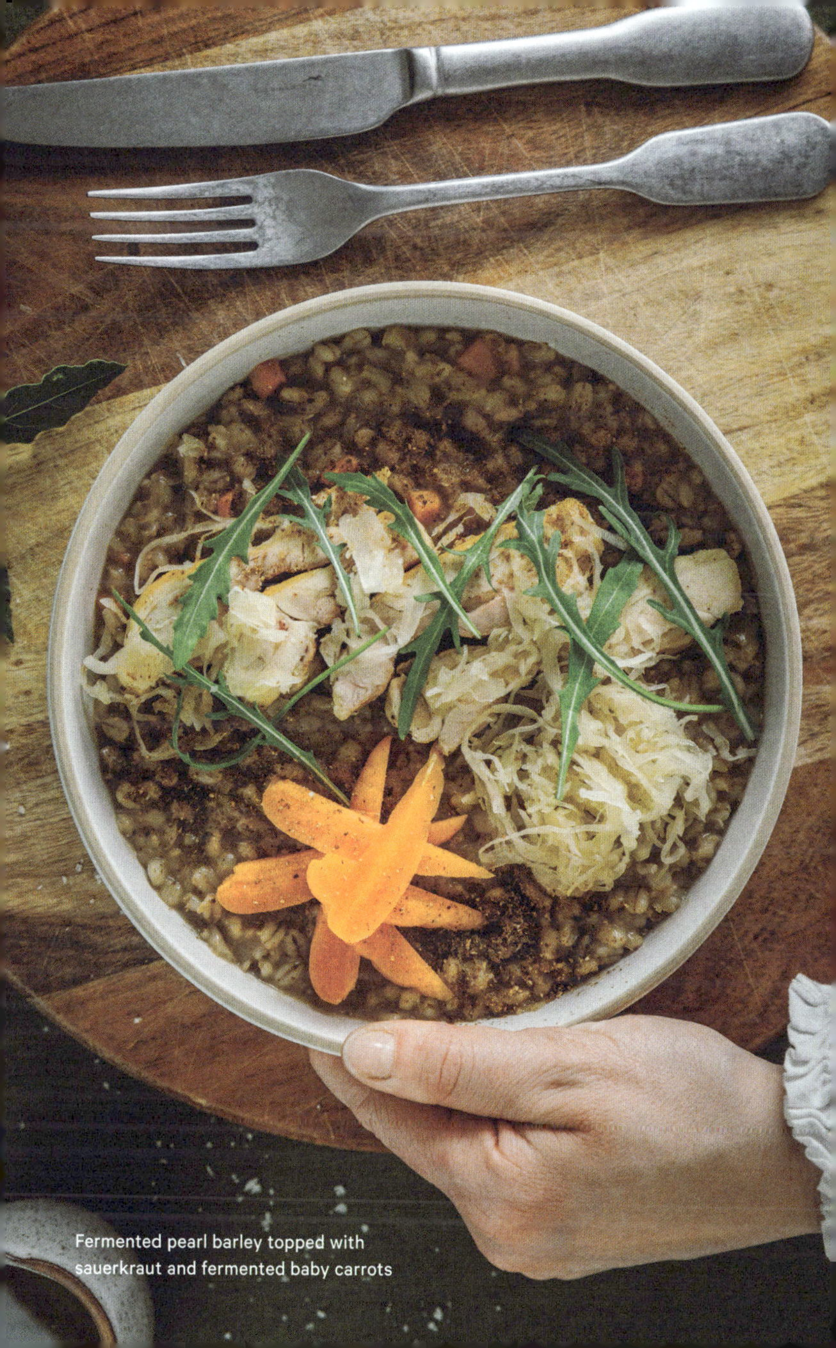

Fermented pearl barley topped with sauerkraut and fermented baby carrots

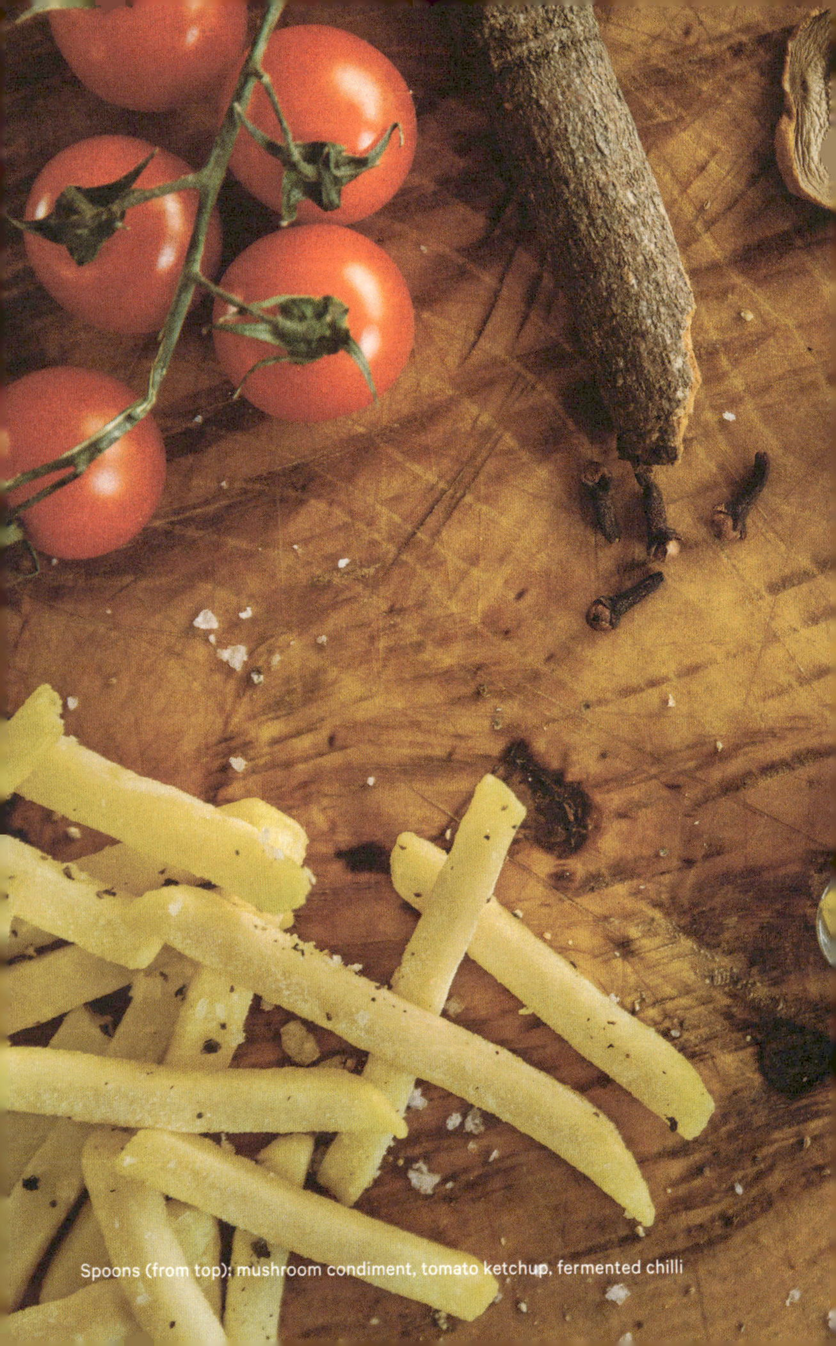

Spoons (from top): mushroom condiment, tomato ketchup, fermented chilli

5
Condiments and other fermented sauces

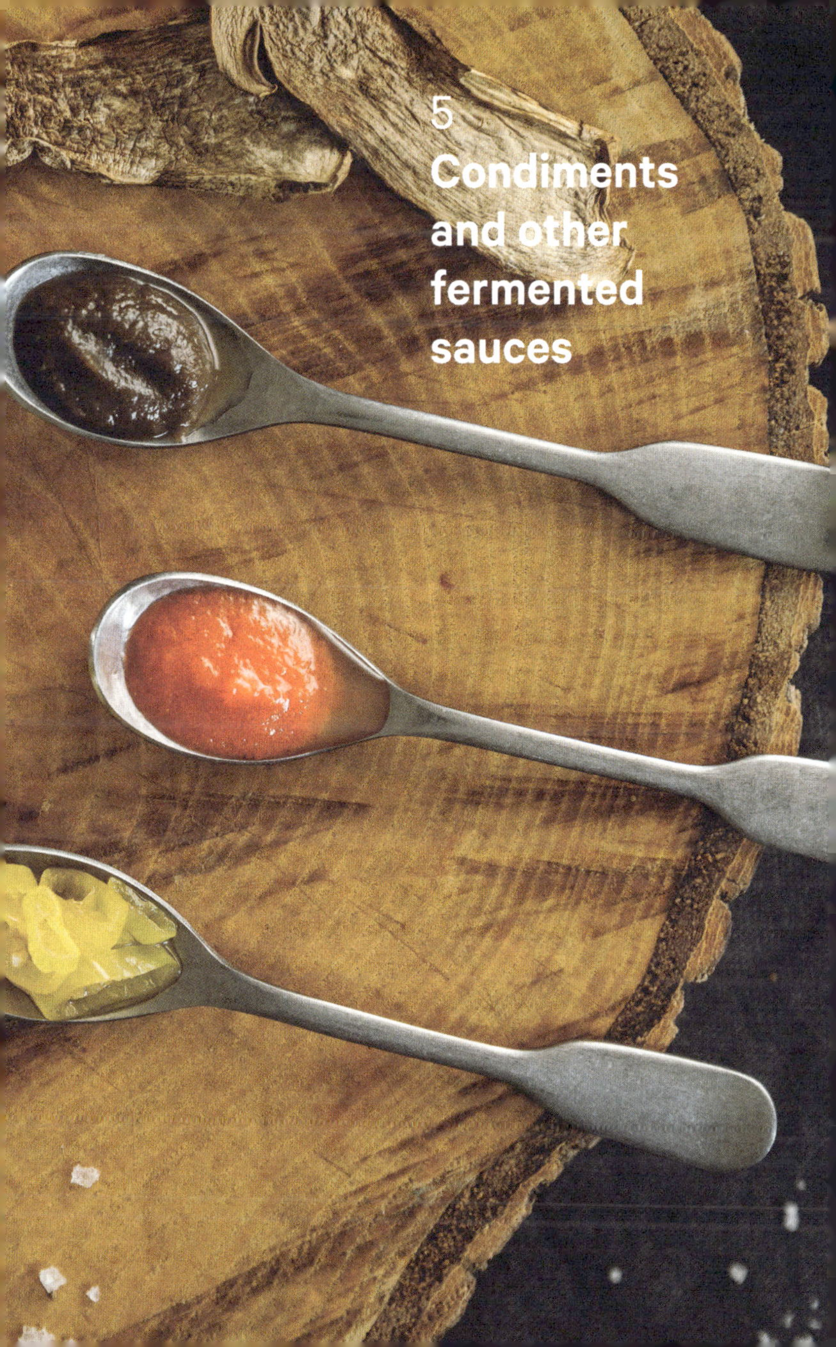

Fermented tomato ketchup and fermented tomato water

If you're anything like us, the idea of sprinkling sugar on your chips, French fries or any fried potato side might seem odd. Yet here we are, living in a world where tomato ketchup — a universal staple — has crept up in sugar content and barely contains any tomatoes. But what if you could have the tangy essence of tomatoes without the cloying sweetness? Imagine a condiment that brings bold umami, moreish acidity and savoury satisfaction, one that is live in probiotics and classified as a healthy food.

This is a two-product recipe: one that kids and adults love (ketchup) and one that's definitely for adults (tomato water). Chilled tomato-water summer soups make us giddy when the best of the greenhouse produce comes through in late summer. Traditionally made by chopping and salting tomatoes, then hanging them in cheesecloth and catching the clear liquid, tomato water is the stuff of kitchen lore and has plenty of uses. It leaves a by-product of tomato pulp and seeds that we thought might convert into ketchup. We tried many different ways — to cut a long story short, we found that fermenting the tomatoes from the start was the most straightforward and successful process.

This method takes tomato water into another dimension, while also creating a fridge-stable ketchup free from sugar. Win-win. Choose the best tomatoes you can find; in a perfect world, that would be end-of-the-summer-season heritage or heirloom varieties with green vine stalks, which we add for that nostalgic greenhouse scent. Feel free to use a mixture of tomatoes.

KIT: *Tessellating tubs, drawstring spice bag or muslin cloth (optional), funnel, 2 x 500ml (17fl oz) sauce bottles*

—

1kg (2lb 4oz) vine-on tomatoes
natural sea salt
1 cinnamon stick
1 tsp whole allspice berries
2 bay leaves
1 black cardamom pod
¼ tsp celery seeds
1 clove
¼ tsp cumin seeds
10 white whole peppercorns

Part 1: Fermenting the tomatoes

Retaining the green vine stalks, slice the tomatoes through their middles to expose the seeds and pulp. Over a bowl, pull the seeds free — don't be afraid to poke your fingers inside the tomato cavity as you go, catching the seeds and juices in the bowl.

Weigh the seed pulp and calculate 1% of that quantity to work out how much salt you need. For instance, 200g (7oz) × 0.01 = 2g (scant ½ tsp) salt. Stir this through to dissolve the salt, then transfer the pulp to a sieve set over a bowl. The action of the salt will draw the moisture from around the seeds over time.

We recommend using the tessellating tub method to make this recipe. As we are using vine fruits, kahm yeast will be present, so we want to do our best to minimise its growth (see page 48). The tessellating tubs will also apply a little pressure to keep the tomato wedges compressed and tomato water running free. Make a note of the weight of your tub and write this number on the outside.

Put the deseeded tomato halves into the tub with the vine stalks and cinnamon stick. Put all the remaining spices into a spice bag or tie them in a square of muslin cloth and add this to the tub. Alternatively you can just chuck them in whole and strain them out later. We think this spice blend gives excellent results, but you can create your own and use ground spice if that is what you have; just use a little less.

Add the tomato liquid that has drained to the tub but leave the tomato seeds to continue draining overnight. Add any further juice to the batch the following day. The tomato seeds can be dried and planted next year.

Weigh up the total and calculate the required 2% salt and stir this through the mixture. Before adding the second tessellating tub, add a cling film layer between them to prevent the formation of kahm yeast.

Ferment on the worktop for 2–3 weeks, paying attention to how the bubbling slows over time. Taste the tomato water as it develops over time. Ahhhh...mazing.

Part 2: Extracting the tomato water

When fermentation is complete, remove the spice bag. Set a sieve over a large bowl and pour in your mixture, allowing it to drain. Once most of the liquid has passed through, transfer everything left in the sieve — including the softened tomato skins — to a blender. Blend until smooth, creating a reddish-pink sauce. This is your ketchup.

Transfer to a suitable sauce bottle, label and date and store in the fridge. See pages 50–51 for storing longer than 1 month.

SERVE WITH: *You don't need us to tell you how to use tomato ketchup...*

(continued overleaf)

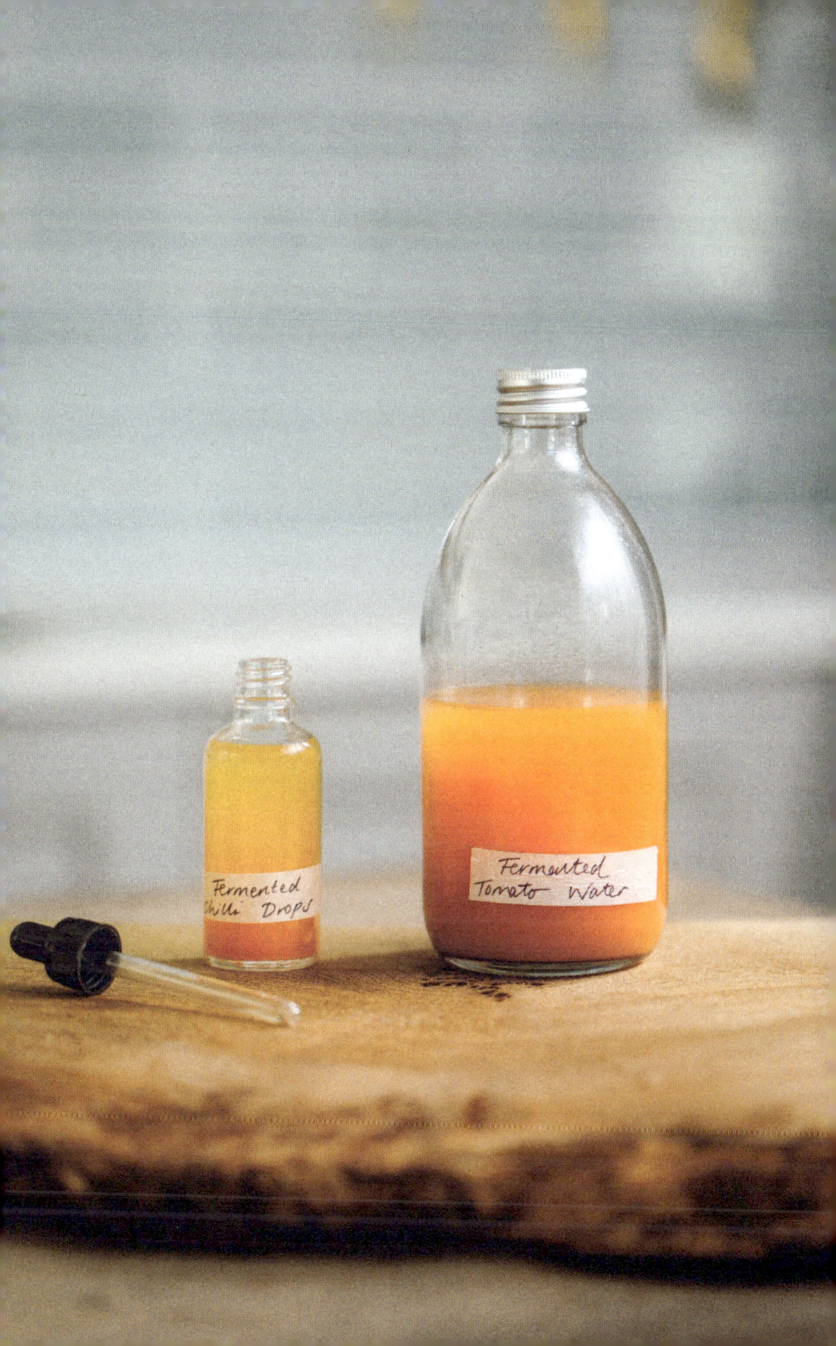
Fermented
Chilli Drops
Fermented
Tomato Water

Now, back to the liquid in the bowl—this is your fermented tomato water. Fermented tomato water holds the crown as the most grown-up, delicious liquid on which we've set our taste buds. Although technically a 'by-product' of the ketchup above, we have found a couple of wonderful ways to use it:

A chilled 'soup' starter

Finely slice courgettes, cut tomatoes into segments and tear basil leaves, then add a small handful of each to individual bowls. Dust with nigella seeds and drizzle with olive oil. Finally, pour a little of the tomato water over to serve. A quick-to-make late-summer showstopper!

Fermented sangrita and tequila

Here we've paired sangrita (a miniature Virgin Mary) with quality tequila. Taking alternate sips of these two drinks is a truly otherworldly experience. For one person, mix 30ml (2 tbsp) fermented tomato water with 20ml (1½ tbsp) orange juice and a dash of Tabasco or a few fermented chilli drops (see page 108). Pour this into one small glass, then pour 50ml (3 tbsp) blue agave tequila into another small glass. Sip first one, then the other and continue to take alternating sips. Salut!

Mushroom condiment

Mushrooms are very high in umami compounds. Umami is often described as the 'fifth taste' and is found in foods like aged cheese, tomatoes, mushrooms and soy sauce. Because they are already high in umami moreish-ness, we can harness this to make a very simple-to-prepare condiment and stock.

Before starting this recipe, you will need some liquid from a previous ferment or brine ferment to use as a 'starter'. Mushrooms have less lactobacillus present because they've had a life growing in the dark, so adding a tablespoon or two of sauerkraut juice will kick-start the mixture to success.

KIT: *Clip-top jar or tessellating tubs, high-speed blender, 200ml (7fl oz) sauce bottle*

—

400–500g (14–18oz) chestnut mushrooms
natural sea salt
1–2 tbsp 'starter' from another ferment
dash of apple cider vinegar

Slice the mushrooms. Place your chosen fermentation vessel on the scales and set to zero. Add the mushrooms and half of their weight in water. (Mushrooms are 70 per cent water, and they will give up that liquid when the salt arrives.) Make a note of the total weight and calculate the amount of salt needed at 2%. Add the salt, plus the 'starter'.

Before closing the lid or adding the second tessellating tub, add a cling film layer to prevent the formation of kahm yeast (see page 48). Place on the work surface and allow to ferment for 3 weeks, keeping an eye on the acidity level as the days and weeks progress.

When fermentation is complete, strain the mushrooms, retaining the brine, then add to a high-speed blender with a splash of the fermenting brine to loosen, and blend to a smooth consistency. Season with a dash of apple cider vinegar then add to a sauce bottle. Label, date and refrigerate (see pages 50–51).

SERVE WITH: *This works in the same way as a ketchup or brown sauce. It's delighted to be on a fry-up, but also elegant enough to go with steak and similarly grilled meats.*

The brine, kept refrigerated, can be used as a base for soups —it works as a natural flavour enhancer for anywhere a recipe calls for stock. Risotto is a place that thrives with its inclusion.

Chilli sauce and fermented chilli drops

Chilli peppers come in a vast range of spiciness, usually measured in Scoville heat units (SHU). For example, a bell pepper is 0 SHU, jalapeños are 2,500–8,000 SHU, while the fearsome Carolina Reaper is over 2 million SHU.

Chilli sauce is very well suited to fermentation. The heat gets rounded off somewhat and the fermentation process coaxes out many flavour compounds that chilli peppers have alongside their fiery capsaicin. Simple to produce and easy to blend with complementary herbs and spices, you'll also get two products from one when fermenting: a blended hot sauce and the liquid left behind, which we call chilli drops. It's similar to Tabasco and can be dotted on any food where you'd like more heat.

KIT: *Clip-top jar or tessellating tubs, high-speed blender, funnel, 2 × 250ml (9fl oz) sauce bottles*

100g (3½oz) fresh chillies, sliced and deseeded
300g (10½oz) red, yellow or green bell peppers (of a similar colour to your chillies), sliced and deseeded
4 garlic cloves, sliced
¼ tsp cumin seeds
¼ tsp celery seeds
a dash of apple cider vinegar

Place your fermentation vessel on the scales and set to zero. Add all the ingredients and top with water, until just submerged. Take note of the total weight and calculate the amount of salt needed at 2%.

Before closing the lid or adding the second tessellating tub, add a cling film layer to prevent the formation of kahm yeast (see page 48) as we're dealing with vine-like plants here. Allow to ferment for 3–4 weeks.

When fermentation has stopped, brave a taste. It'll be spicy but not wild. Strain the solids and set aside the liquid brine. Blend the solids in a high-speed blender, adding a splash of chilli brine if loosening is required. Bottle, label and date.

The clear-ish, light-hued brine left over is your fermented 'chilli drops'. To ensure this ferment has a long life, add a dash of 6% acidity vinegar. Raw unpasteurised apple cider vinegar is ideal, look for 'with mother' or 'live' on the bottle. Store in a bottle, refrigerate and use where you'd usually use Tabasco. See pages 50–51 for storing your chilli sauce and chilli drops for longer than 1 month.

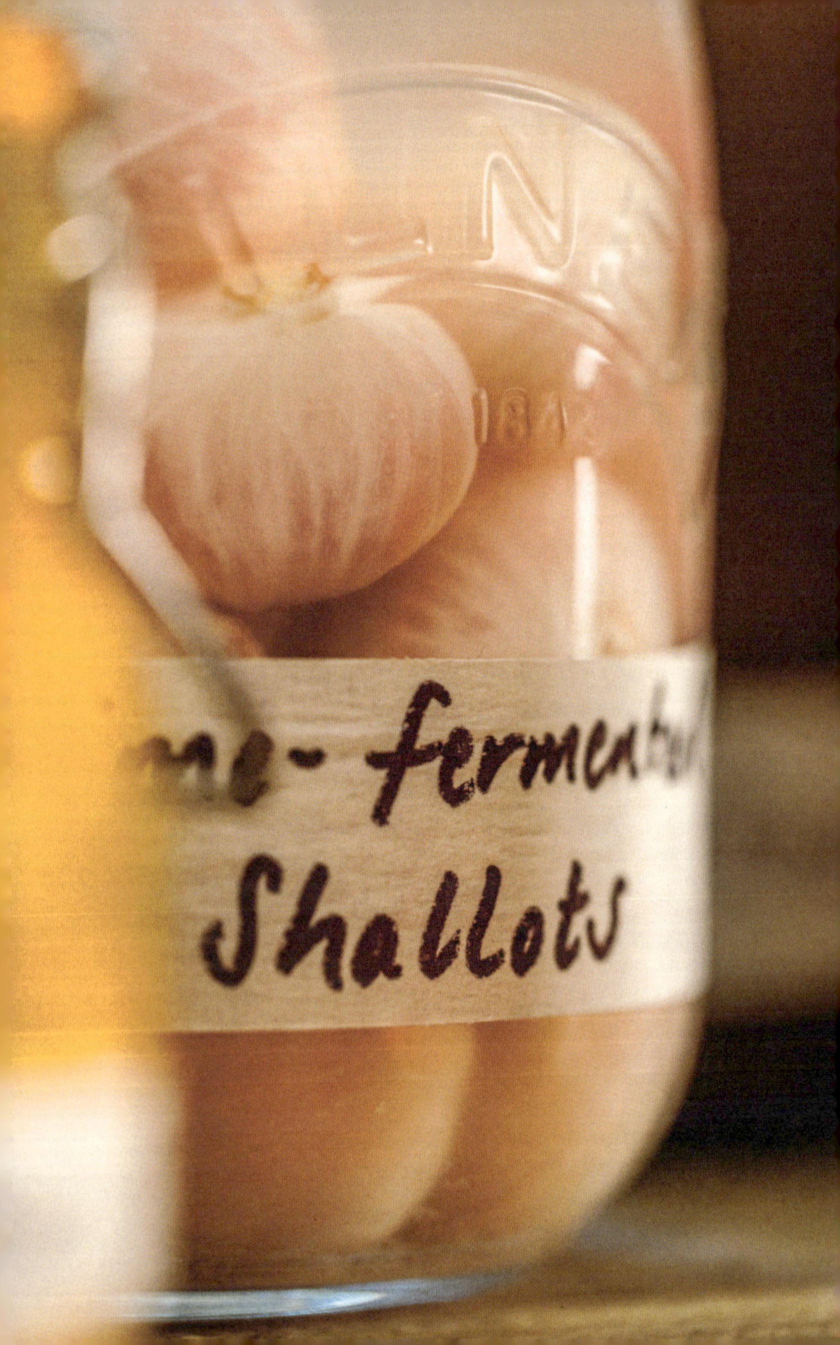
Shallots

Lime-fermented shallots

When you rescue and transform food that might ordinarily end up as compost, it is truly thrilling. The clever Indian soul who made the first batch of lime chutney would have had a proud smile for years to come. Let us make lime-fermented shallots and then use the discarded lime peels to make lime 'pickle' — see next recipe!

We've designed these two recipes to work off the supermarket shelf. In our local shop, one bag of small shallot onions is 500g (1lb 2oz), and good Brazilian limes come in nets of five. We end up with about 1kg (2lb 4oz) jar of crisp, not-pickled-but fermented shallots and precisely 500g (1lb 2oz) of fermented lime 'pickle'. Excellent! Shop for the spices at the same time to ensure you can make both recipes together.

KIT: *Clip-top jar or tessellating tubs, hand juicer*

—

500g (1lb 2oz) shallots, small round variety
10 limes, cut into halves or eights depending on your juicer
natural sea salt

Lightly top and tail the shallots and peel them, making sure you've removed all the skins. Peeling is fiddly, but all good things come with a challenge. Juice the limes and keep the skins.

Place your fermentation vessel on the scales and set to zero. Add the peeled shallots and lime juice and cover with water until the shallots are fully submerged. Note the final weight, calculate the salt content to — yes, you guessed it — 2% and add it.

Cover with a layer of cling film, close the lid (or place your second tessellating tub on top of the first), and wish it well. Because the acidity starts high from the lime juice and we are using whole shallots, it can take longer to ferment; allow 4–6 weeks. Keep a close eye to see if the bubbling of the onions has stopped. This is your indication that fermentation is complete. If using tubs, transfer to a jar. Label your jar with the date, and store it in the fridge.

SERVE WITH: *An integral part of a ploughman's lunch — a humble serving of Cheddar cheese, bread, pickle and of course, a fermented rather than 'pickled' shallot.*

These lime-scented shallots are magic for lifting dishes where cream and fish are cooked together. Finely slice or dice to garnish to give an acidic zip and cut through the cream.

Fermented lime 'pickle'

> **The art of fermentation is the art of patience.**
> Sandor Katz

Patience is undoubtedly required for this one, partly because this ferment takes a while to get a wriggle on. However, it's very long-lived. We've known jars that have lasted two house moves and are still perfect. We're talking years good!

KIT: *500ml (17fl oz) clip-top jar*

—

discarded lime wedges from the previous recipe
1 tsp ground turmeric
¼ tsp asafoetida

1 tsp Kashmiri chilli powder
natural sea salt
1 tbsp 'starter' from another ferment

For the toasting mix
1 tsp mustard seeds
1 tsp fennel seeds
⅛ tsp fenugreek seeds
½ tsp nigella seeds

Start by toasting the seeds for the toasting mix in a dry frying pan over a medium heat until they start to pop and release all the luscious scents. Remove from the heat and allow to cool.

Chop the discarded lime wedges — eighths is about right. Place a bowl on the scales and set to zero, then tip in all the chopped limes, ground spices and toasting mix. It'll add up to something random, like 545g (19oz). As always, we want to add 2% salt.

Combine and mix the ingredients and salt well. Add the starter liquid from another ferment, then pack the mix into the jar tightly. Add a layer of cling film, and bid it farewell for 4–6 weeks. The pH can register as low as 2.5 in the long term. It is as safe as it gets.

SERVE WITH: *In the UK, lime pickle is eaten as an appetiser with poppadoms and raita before an Indian curry. Even the thought of its unusual, sour, bitter and hot tones can make you salivate in anticipation. It is one of the world's most unique tastes and worth being patient to try.*

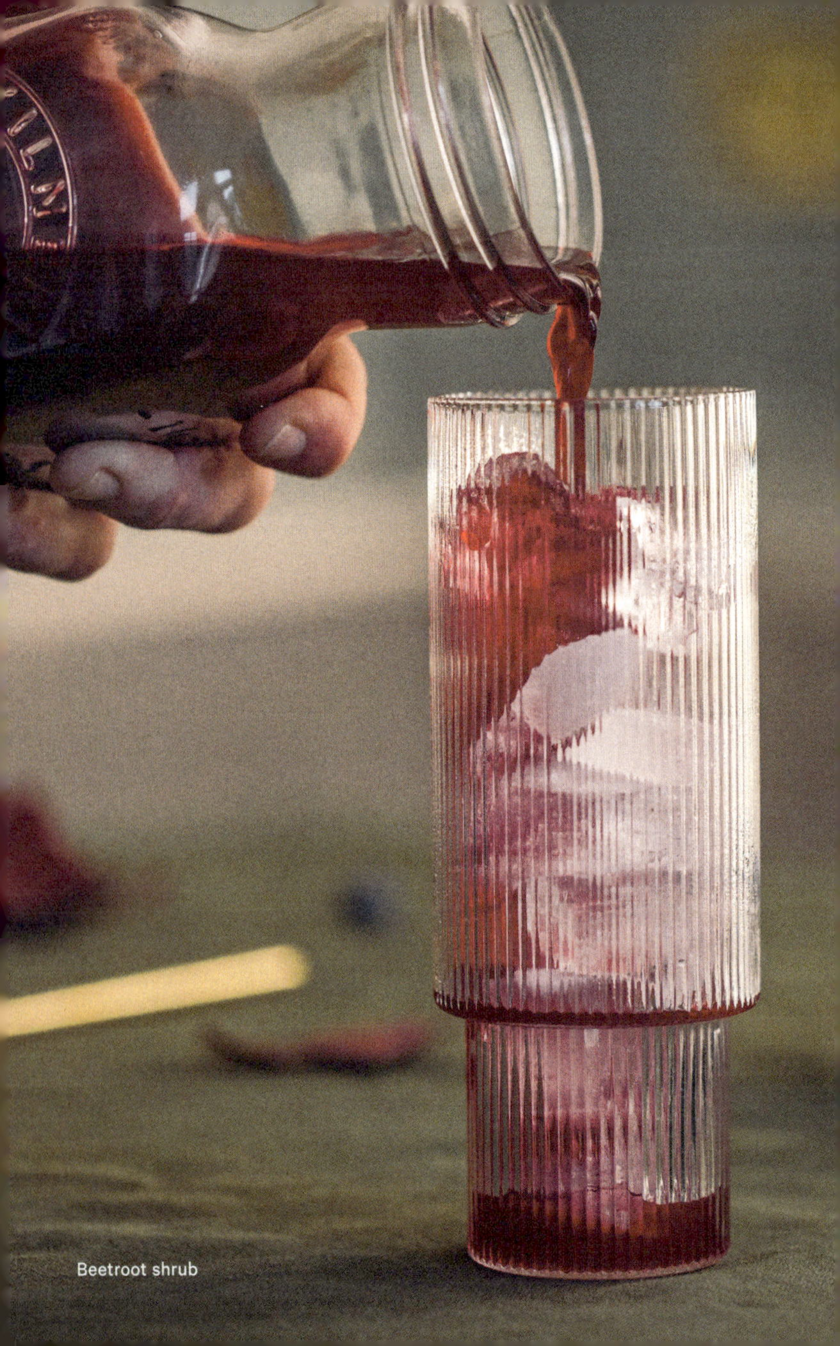

Beetroot shrub

6
Wild sodas and fermented drinks

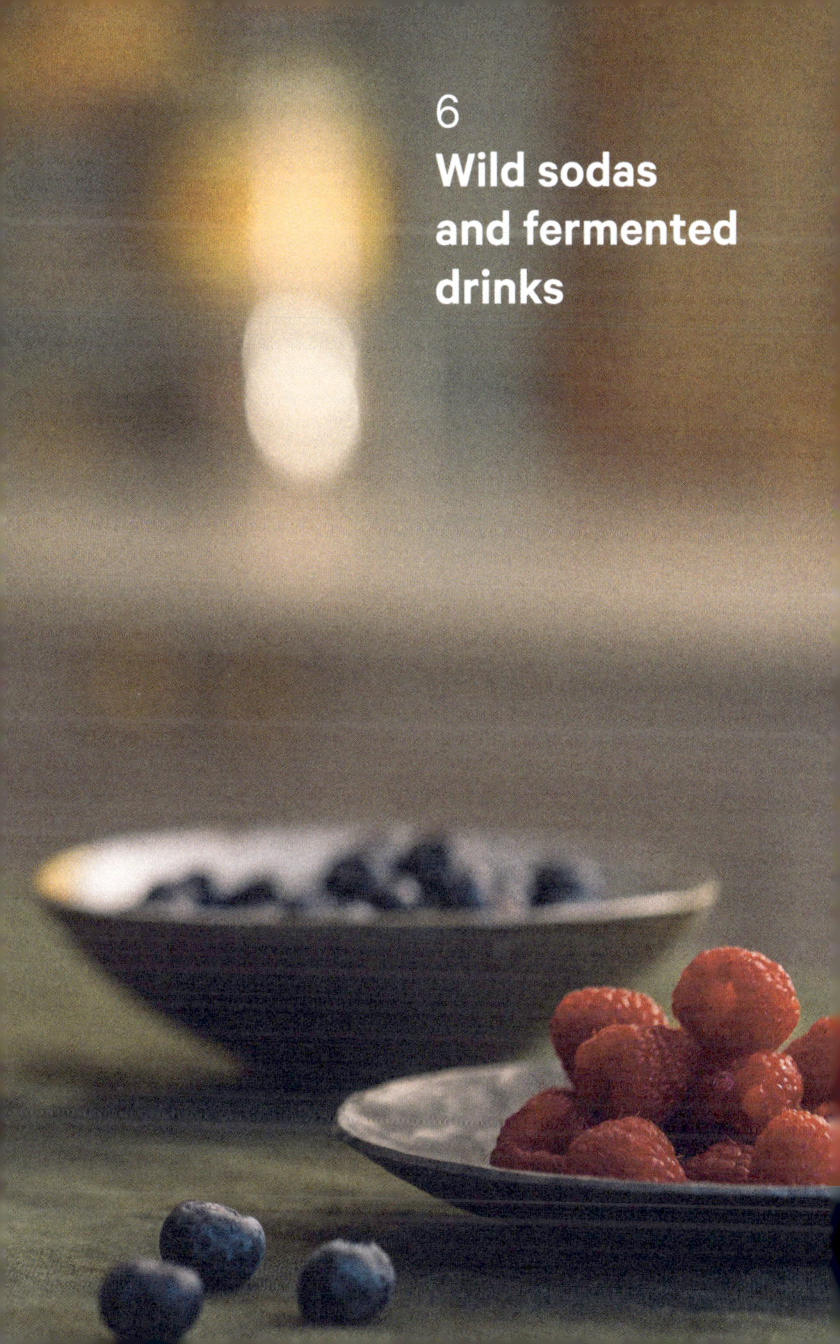

Fermented drinks are full of probiotic microbes, vitamins, minerals and antioxidants, all of which are great for our health. Incorporating fermented drinks into our diet is a wonderful way of benefiting from those nutrients. We've mastered some delicious and simple recipes to make and take care of, ensuring you can fit them into your busy schedules.

Fermented drinks offer endless flavour combinations, allowing you to use what you have. We like to work with the seasons, ensuring ingredients are at their peak in terms of flavour and freshness, reducing waste and keeping our larder and fridge interesting year-round.

Some of the drinks here are fermented using a SCOBY, or 'symbiotic culture of bacteria and yeast'. SCOBYs can take the form of a cellulose disc (such as in kombucha or vinegar) or gelatinous 'grains' (used to make milk and water kefir). See the Resources (page 151) for recommended suppliers.

Kombucha (fermented black or green tea) can be tricky to maintain, much like the care and attention that sourdough bread requires. Kombucha is sometimes more sensitive to environmental factors like temperature, pH and oxygen levels. For this reason, we've opted to focus on recipes for fermented drinks which are simpler and easy to build into your weekly routine.

Other ways of making fermented drinks involve using yeasts (such as in our pine needle soda, tepache and kvass). Yeasts can be found naturally on plants and fruits; we call these wild yeasts. They can also be manufactured (such as those used in beer and winemaking).

The sugars present at the start are predominantly metabolised after fermentation, leaving you with low-sugar drinks — fantastic substitutes for many soft drinks on the market. They're also great in cocktails; we often use our kefir water or fermented sodas instead of tonic in a G&T! See the end of the chapter for our favourite cocktail recommendations using ferments.

Best containers for fermented drinks

Plastic bottles that have housed carbonated drinks are helpful to the home fermenter as they are pressure-resistant and inexpensive. If you'd prefer not to use plastic, a tall glass bottle or jar with a screw-top lid — left on loosely — is the way. Essentially, you want a vessel that withstands the pressure or allows a little gas to escape to avoid any minor explosions! You can use round glass clip-top bottles, as long as you remember to regularly 'burp' them to let gas escape. Steer clear of any clip-top square glass bottles; they're the most volatile!

Water kefir

This is a wonderful yet simple fermented drink to make. It has a slight effervescence to it and is made using water kefir grains, which are a type of SCOBY. The bacteria and yeasts in the grains break down the sugars in the liquid and ferment, giving off carbon dioxide, responsible for the fizz. It's an excellent low-sugar drink for children or if you're starting your fermentation journey, as it tastes much less tart than kombucha. This basic recipe uses lemon for a light, refreshing taste similar to lemonade.

Once fermented, it can be strained and bottled as is or flavoured in an optional 'secondary fermentation' (without the grains) with fruit, berries or herbs — see the end of the recipe for our favourite flavour combinations. Secondary fermentation is also a great way of using up fruit or vegetable scraps.

Buy grains from any reputable fermenting supplier; the grains will arrive either dehydrated or in a sugar solution. We prefer the ones in a solution if available.

In optimum conditions, your kefir grains will multiply. As they increase in weight, you'll need to increase the measurements of water and sugar to compensate. Alternatively, gift your excess grains to a friend / family member or pop them on your compost. If you want a break from making water kefir, are going away on holiday, or your grains have multiplied, you can 'sleep' some of them temporarily. To do this, you'll want to store them in a screw-top jar in the fridge in a water / sugar solution (the same method as when making the kefir water, but with slightly different ratios). Using a higher amount of sugar, plus the colder temperature, will allow you to keep the grains like this for a few weeks. For every tablespoon of grains you want to store, you'll need 60ml (4 tablespoons) of water, and 15g (1 tablespoon) of sugar dissolved in the water. Don't screw the jar lid on tightly—you'll want a bit of gas to be able to escape. Pop in the fridge and store for up to 4 weeks. Water kefir grains do not respond well to freezing. And remember, if you live in an area where water is treated with chlorine, it's best to use filtered water or water that's been boiled and left to cool to room temperature.

KIT: *Glass clip-top jar with a rubber seal, large enough to leave some air when filled, funnel, sieve, container for storing kefir once made (see page 117)*

water kefir grains
water
golden caster sugar / unrefined sugar
½ lemon (optional)
1 organic (unsulphured) dried apricot or fig (optional)

Measure out your grains to see how many tablespoons you have, then decide how much water kefir you want to make. For every tablespoon of grains, you'll need 15g (1 tablespoon) sugar and 250ml (1 cup) water.

Boil the water, and once it's cooled slightly, pour it into a clean clip-top jar. Add the sugar and mix until it dissolves.

Allow to cool fully to room temperature, then add your grains, plus your halved lemon and a dried apricot or fig, if using. (The dried fruit contains minerals and nutrients that help the grains develop. Add it to your ferment if you want to increase the growth of your grains or after a period of 'sleep' to kick-start the fermentation process again.)

Clip the lid on and leave it out on the kitchen work surface in a spot that won't get direct sunlight. After 24 hours, the mixture should start to fizz. Each day, 'burp' the kefir by releasing the lid slightly to let out some gas. You want to get it to a sweet spot where the sugar content has reduced, and there's a lovely effervescence, but it's not too dry. The best way to achieve this is to taste it daily — you'll start to notice the changes. The process should take roughly 2–3 days, depending on the time of year and the temperature inside your house. The warmer it is, the faster fermentation usually happens. We've found that in a room around 16–18°C (60–64°F), a batch of 1 litre (4 cups) of kefir takes about 3 days to ferment, which sits pretty well with the speed at which we drink it as a household of two people.

After 3 days, or once you've reached your desired taste / fizziness, strain the kefir water into your container. A time-effective method we use is to put a funnel into the mouth of a bottle and pop a small sieve into the funnel, skipping the need for a jug. Your water kefir will taste light, refreshing and lemony — refrigerate now, or if secondary fermenting, follow the next step.

Optional secondary fermentation / flavouring

You can now add more flavour to your kefir water. Once bottled or in your vessel of choice, add a handful of chopped fruit, berries, raw vegetables, herbs or botanicals to flavour it. Then, leave it out on the counter to ferment for another day before refrigerating. The possible flavour combinations are limitless, but we have some tried-and-tested favourites: Rhubarb and orange, Ginger and thyme, Elderflower, Rose, Hibiscus, Blackcurrant, Raspberry and peppercorn, Strawberry and basil, Cucumber and mint, Beetroot and cinnamon.

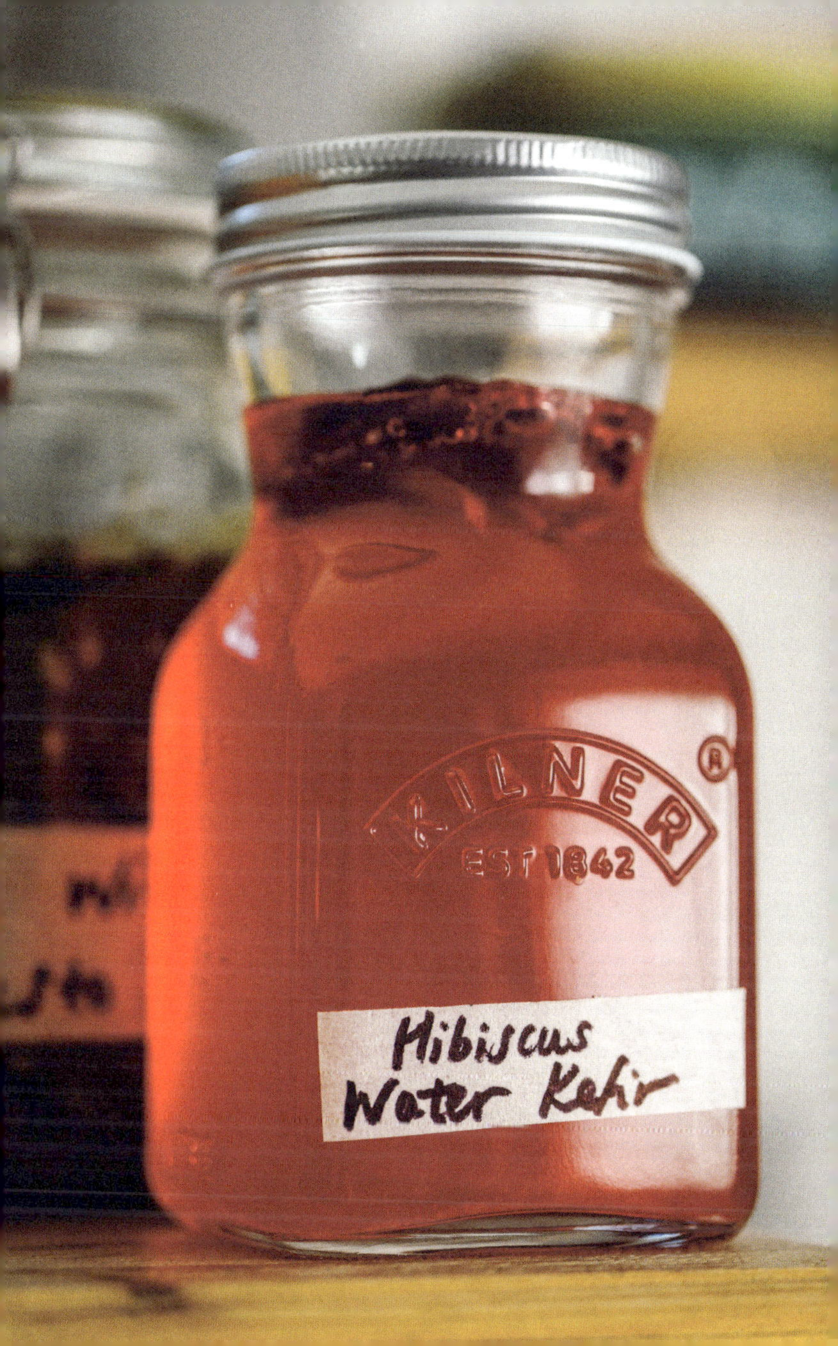
KILNER
EST 1842
Hibiscus
Water Kefir

Milk kefir

Milk kefir is a fermented milk drink made using milk kefir grains, a type of SCOBY. Note that these are different from water kefir grains; milk kefir grains are white (see image on page 124), whereas water kefir grains are clear. They each feed off different things and produce distinct ferments.

When put into milk and left for roughly 24 hours, milk kefir grains convert lactose into lactic acid and create an environment where harmful bacteria (the ones which turn milk 'off') cannot survive. Just as with yoghurt making, this is why it's perfectly safe to ferment your milk at room temperature with regular and proper care and upkeep. Cold temperatures can harm the growth of the microbes essential for this process, so as much as possible, avoid fermenting milk kefir in a fridge.

Making milk kefir doesn't take long (mere minutes), but it is a daily task. If you get into the habit of checking, straining and bottling every 24 hours, it will soon become a part of your daily routine. We like to do this after dinner — that way we can flavour and bottle our freshly made kefir and pop it into the fridge then it's nice and cold, ready for breakfast the following morning.

Milk kefir grains can be found from reputable fermentation suppliers. They'll arrive in a little sachet or pouch, sometimes in a bit of milk. Once you have your grains, you'll need to start off making on a small scale and gradually build your batches up with larger amounts of milk each time.

Add milk kefir to smoothies, eat instead of yoghurt with granola or muesli, or drink as it is. The tangy flavour of milk kefir can be an acquired taste. If you'd like to make it a little more palatable, try popping a piece of lemon peel in your finished product overnight or add a few drops of vanilla extract. You can also swirl in some honey or fruit compote before drinking.

Aftercare

Much like water kefir grains, milk kefir grains will grow and reproduce in a happy environment. You want to ensure the bacteria and yeasts have adequate food. When you find your grains growing in size and weight, you'll need to increase the amount of milk you're adding, or if you're happy with the amount of kefir you are already producing, gift some grains to a friend. If you want to store the spare grains, freezing works well. Take the grains, pop them into a small ziplock bag or pot, and transfer them to the freezer. When it comes to waking the grains up again to use, remember that it may take a few days for them to come alive again. Follow the same process below but be patient! If you are heading on holiday or want to take a break from making kefir, you can temporarily store them in the fridge for up to 3 weeks by putting them in a ratio of 1:20 grains to milk. For 5g (1 tsp) grains, use 100ml (scant ½ cup) milk.

KIT: *A selection of clean jars of various sizes (screw or clip-top), funnel, sieve, a container / jar / bottle to store your finished product in once made*

—

milk kefir grains
milk (preferably full-fat and organic)
optional flavours (lemon peel, vanilla extract)

To start from scratch with new grains, we advise building up in the following stages.

Take the smallest of your jars, place your grains inside and cover with milk. Start with a ratio of 1:10. For example, if your grains weigh 5g, the amount of milk at this stage needs to be about 50ml (3½ tablespoons). The aim is to have no more than a 2 cm (¾ in) gap at the top of the jar; the grains seem to prefer it this way. Clip or screw the lid onto the jar and leave on the kitchen work surface for 12 hours.

Check to see if the milk has set. You're looking for a thick layer on the surface, similar to yoghurt. It will also smell slightly sour and tangy. If there are no signs of action, put the lid back on and leave for another 6–12 hours.

Once the milk has set, spoon out the grains or strain through a sieve. Shake the sieve gently to run the liquid through so that you don't risk crushing and damaging the grains. Throw away this initial batch — it won't harm you, but it won't taste right yet.

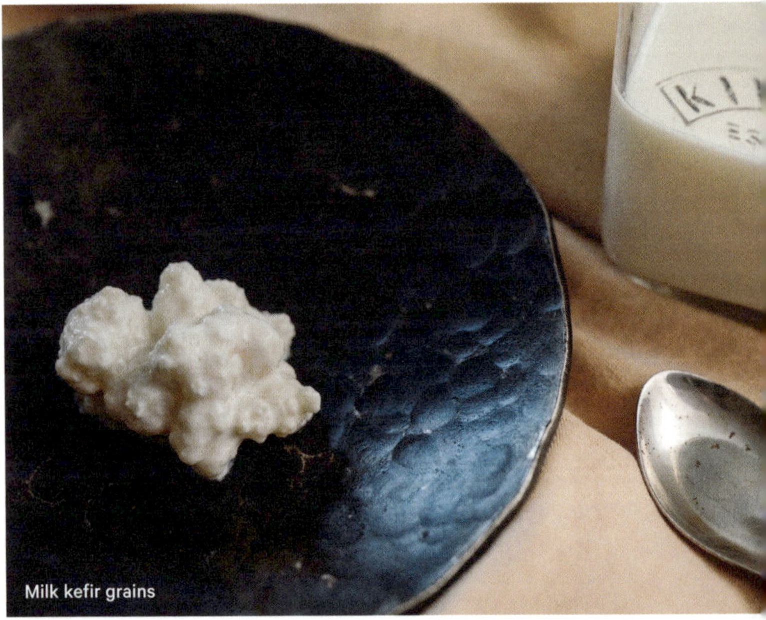

Milk kefir grains

Repeat the process with the same measurements. This time, you can drink the finished product or bottle and store it in the fridge. Flavour the bottled kefir if you like.

With the third batch, you can start to scale up. Try the grains in 100ml (scant ½ cup) milk this time. Use a slightly larger jar if you need — just keep a 2 cm (¾ in) gap at the top of the jar.

Keep scaling up gradually if you like; your 5g grains will make up to about 1 litre (4 cups) of kefir quite happily. We'd recommend scaling up in 100ml (scant ½ cup) increments. See the aftercare section on page 123 for what to do when your grains grow in size.

Your finished kefir will keep in the fridge for a couple of weeks, although you'll likely drink it before this point. As it takes so little time to ferment and requires daily bottling, aim to make just what you and your household consume. There's no need to create and store large batches unless you plan to gift them.

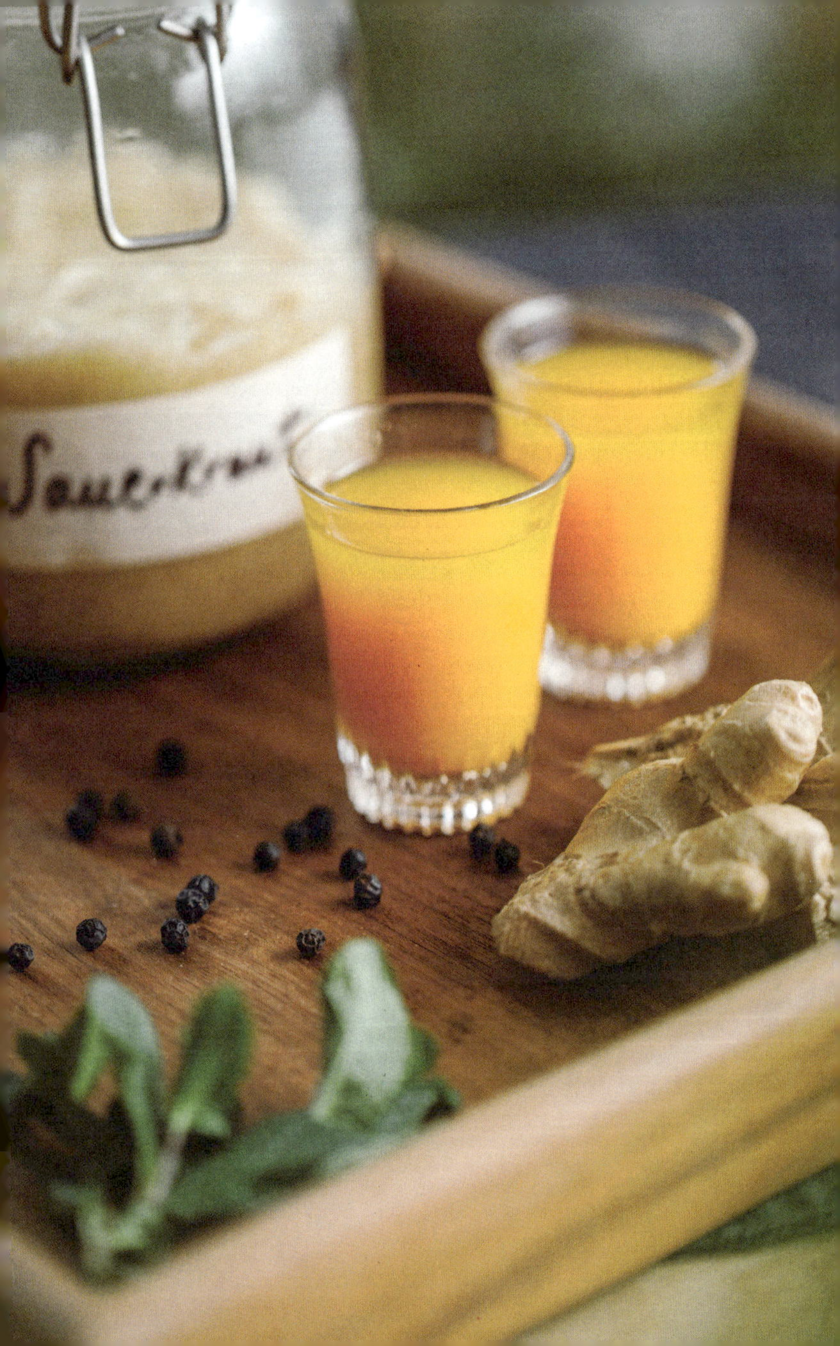

Sauerkraut brine gut shots

Once you've made and consumed a batch of sauerkraut, you'll be left with the brine—rich in probiotics and beneficial bacteria that our gut flora thrives on. Rather than throw it away, we've found a great way to use this liquid gold—in gut shots! These are super-simple to make, and you can swap in or out with other flavours, depending on your tastes or what you have to use up at the bottom of the fridge and fruit bowl.

Take a 50ml (2fl oz) shot daily, on its own, or in a smoothie or juice. It's a brilliant way to start the day—the fiery flavour and citrus fruit really wake you up and get you going!

KIT: *High-speed blender (a standard blender will still do the job; it just won't break the mixture down as fine), funnel, sieve, bottle or container to store your brine shots*

150ml (⅔ cup) sauerkraut brine
1 thumb of fresh ginger, peeled and chopped
1 thumb of fresh turmeric, peeled and chopped
juice of 1 lemon
juice of 1 orange
a couple of cracks of black pepper

Blend all your ingredients in a high-speed blender and strain out any pulp through a sieve. Then, bottle it and store it in the fridge for up to a week.

Alternative flavourings

Leafy greens, apples, grapefruit juice, pears, mango, pineapple, garlic (a crowd divider, but an ingredient that's great for your immune system).

Shrubs

Shrubs, also known as drinking vinegars, were traditionally used to preserve fruit and vegetables. However, they have now gained popularity as excellent gut-nourishing drinks. Made using apple cider vinegar and diluted with sparkling or still water, shrubs are a fantastic non-alcoholic beverage and a great alternative to the standard sugar-rich soft drinks on the market. Plus, they are super simple to make!

Shrubs are a great way to use up scraps or gluts — fruit that may be going a little soft, berries on the turn, or peelings you have no use for. They are extremely 'zero-waste' — we use any pulp left over from making our shrubs to make chutney, or as a topping for yoghurt and porridge. As vinegar and sugar are already present, you can just cook the pulp down in a saucepan and store it in the fridge for up to a week.

Research has highlighted many health benefits of regularly consuming raw, unpasteurised apple cider vinegar — studies have shown the probiotics present increase healthy gut bacteria, reduce blood sugar levels and, when consumed before meals, may reduce blood sugar spikes.

Shrubs take this live vinegar and infuse it with the flavour, vitamins and minerals found in fruit or vegetables. This is then sweetened with sugar to make a palatable concentrate suitable for dilution with water or as a fantastic alternative for lemon or lime in cocktails. As a side note, throughout our restaurant's history, we refused to use citrus fruits as an ingredient, instead using creative concoctions such as shrubs to bring that acidic flavour to drink making.

Over the page is one of our favourites, Blackberry and cinnamon, and you'll find more of our flavour suggestions at the end of the recipe. The options are endless — just edit

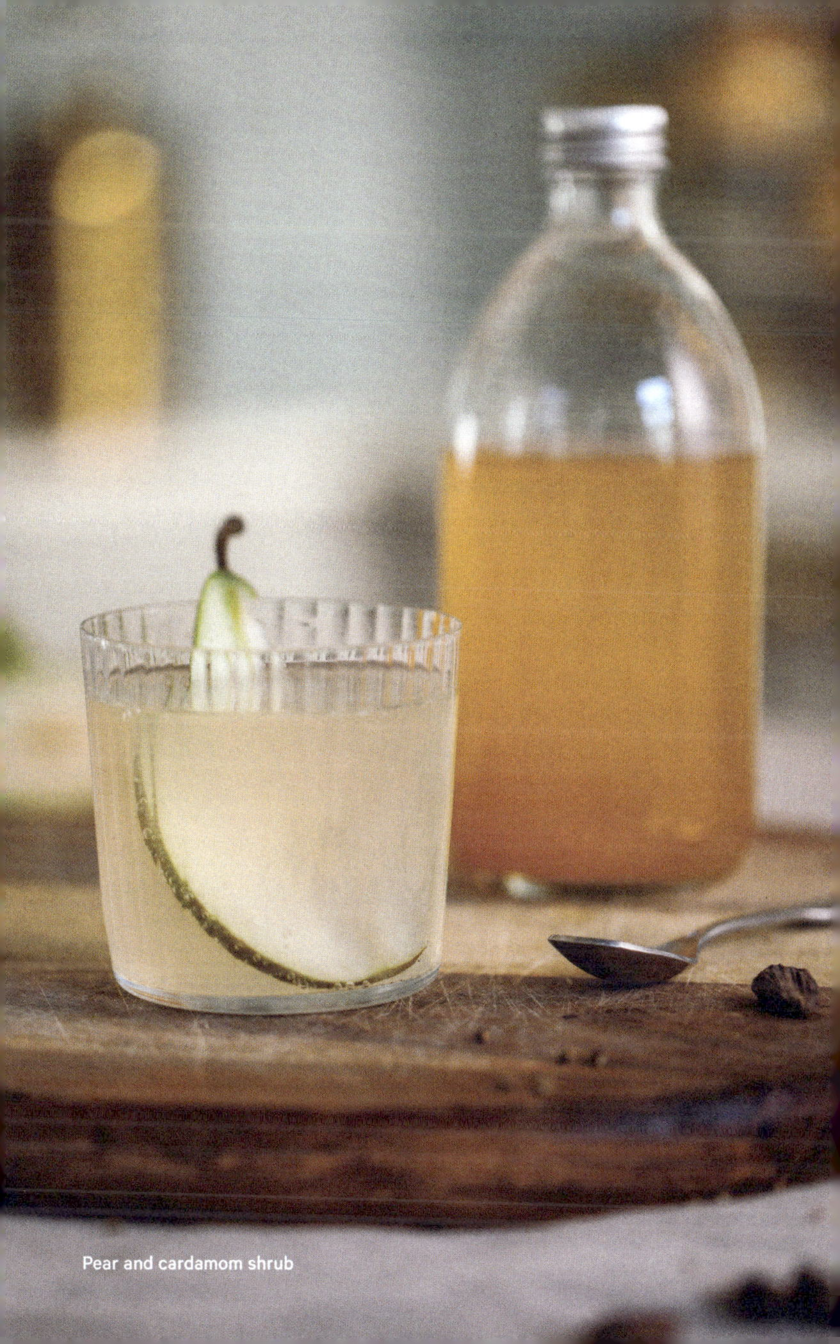

Pear and cardamom shrub

out the fruit or vegetables and choose complementary spices or herbs.

We've found the ratio below to be just the right balance of sugar and acidity. However, you can adjust it to your own taste — if you prefer it less sweet, reduce the amount of sugar you use, or if you like a little more sweetness, increase it.

Aftercare

Once bottled, store it in a cool, dark place. We keep ours in the fridge so they're cold for making cocktails or drinks, but it's not necessary — the apple cider vinegar will keep it preserved. Your shrub will keep for months, even years, but you'll likely drink it before then.

Our ratio uses 1 part fruit or vegetable to 1 part sugar to 2 parts apple cider vinegar. So, for 100g (3½oz) of fruit, you'll need 100g (3½oz) of sugar and 200ml (7fl oz) of apple cider vinegar. The resulting shrub will be slightly more than the amount of apple cider vinegar you use, as liquid will be extracted from the fruit or vegetable, and the sugar will also add some volume. Bear this in mind when selecting a container or bottle to store it in.

Blackberry and cinnamon shrub

KIT: *Jar or tub large enough to hold all your ingredients, funnel, sieve, bottle or container to store your shrub*

—

100g (3½oz) blackberries
100g (3½oz) unrefined cane sugar
1 cinnamon stick (optional)
200ml (7fl oz) raw, unpasteurised apple cider vinegar (look for 'with mother' or 'live' on the bottle)

Combine the blackberries, sugar and cinnamon stick, if using, in a jar or container.

Leave your container in a cool, dark place for about 3 days.* Shake or stir the contents halfway through the process to ensure proper mixing. The fruit or vegetables will start to give off liquid and produce a syrupy consistency. After about 3 days, add the apple cider vinegar to your mixture, stir through and leave for a further 4 days.

After a few days, the vinegar will be infused with all those lovely flavours. Strain the mixture through a sieve to remove the fruit / veg and herbs or spices. Use a funnel to bottle or pour into your container of choice. Labelling your shrub here is good practice, as after making a few different batches, you may forget what flavours you have used!

The remaining fruit or vegetable pulp can be composted, cooked down into a chutney, or used as a topping for granola, yoghurt, porridge, pancakes or desserts.

More shrub flavour ideas

Small berries can be left whole. Chop larger fruits and vegetables into 1 cm (½ in) cubes. Don't forget to remove any stones, pips and stems before chopping if you plan to use the fruit pulp in some way afterwards.

Parsnip and thyme—you can use scrubbed peelings or the actual vegetable here. With a sprig of thyme, it will make a lovely sweet and savoury shrub.

---

* The timings here are flexible; it won't matter if you forget and leave it to infuse for longer. If you know you will be going away for more than 3 or 4 days, just pop it into the fridge before you go. Equally, if you're in a hurry and leave it for a little less time, that's not a problem. We've just found that these timings fit into our schedules and give us the best possible flavour from the ingredients.

Carrot and caraway seed — again, peelings or the body of the vegetable. Combine with ½ teaspoon of caraway seeds per 100g (3½oz) carrots for an earthy anise taste.

Pear and cardamom — lightly crush 3 cardamom pods and add to 100g (3½oz) diced pear.

Plum and burnt bay — chop the plums and remove the stones. Burn the edges of a few bay leaves; they'll crackle and give off a lovely smoky smell. Combined with the sweet plums, this makes a delightfully grown-up-tasting shrub, perfect as an ingredient for cocktails or mocktails.

Strawberry and peppercorn — add ½ tsp peppercorns for the perfect balance of spice with the sweetness of the strawberries.

Peach and honey — swap the sugar for honey in this combination. You can get away with using less honey, as it tastes sweeter than sugar. Try 100g (3½oz) peach, 75g (3oz) honey and 200ml (7fl oz) apple cider vinegar.

Cucumber and mint — classic summer flavours.

Raspberry and rose — you can use wild or garden rose petals; they're all safe to consume, as long as they haven't been sprayed with pesticides. You can also find dried petals in supermarkets. A small handful of petals per 100g (3½oz) raspberries will give a lovely floral flavour.

Beetroot and cumin — use ½ tsp cumin seeds for another tremendously balanced sweet-savoury shrub.

Mango and fig leaf — fig leaves give the most incredible coconut flavour; just chop a leaf into small pieces before mixing with mango and sugar.

Rhubarb and ginger — tart and slightly spicy.

Tepache

Originating from Mexico, tepache is a refreshing fermented drink traditionally made using pineapple peel. It's a great way to use up what would ordinarily be thrown away or composted.

It uses panela (raw cane sugar), though you can also make it with demerara or muscovado sugar. Drink on its own over ice or add a measure of tequila or rum for a boozy alternative on a warm summer's day.

Aftercare

Tepache can be fairly fizzy, so once it's made, store it in a suitable bottle (see page 117) and consume it within a week.

KIT: *Clip-top jar, large enough to leave some air when filled with your solution, funnel, clean piece of muslin, elastic band or string, container for storing your finished tepache*

—

1 litre (4 cups) water
100g (3½oz) panela or brown sugar
1 cinnamon stick
2 star anise
1 thumb of fresh ginger (optional)
peel and core of 1 pineapple

Put the water and sugar into a saucepan and bring to the boil to dissolve the sugar. Let it cool to a lukewarm temperature, then pour it into the clip-top jar, adding the cinnamon stick and other spices.

Add the pineapple peel and core to the sugar solution and ensure it's fully submerged (you may have to wedge some pieces in horizontally to keep them under the surface of the liquid). Cover the top of the jar with the muslin and secure with an elastic band or string. Leave the lid off at this stage.

Pop somewhere warm — an airing cupboard or a shelf next to (but not on top of) a radiator is perfect. Leave for 2 days before removing the muslin and checking on your mixture. By now, the fermentation process should have started, and you'll see froth around the surface. If not, give the mixture a good stir and move it somewhere a little warmer for another couple of days.

After a total of 3–5 days, once you have a decent froth on the surface of the tepache, strain your mixture through a sieve into a bottle or your container of choice and store it in the fridge.

Pine needle soda

This recipe makes an incredible fermented soda, harnessing the natural yeasts found in pine needles. The yeasts feed on the sugar and give off gas, producing a super-fun, fizzy drink that's quick and simple to make. Pine needles have a high vitamin C content, which is excellent for our immune systems. They also have the benefit of being an expectorant (a type of cough medicine) so this is a great drink to make to beat those colds and coughs!

It is crucial to identify and pick from the right tree. Pine trees are a species of conifer or evergreen. Many conifers are edible; however, there are some that are toxic, the most common being the yew tree. We'd recommend checking

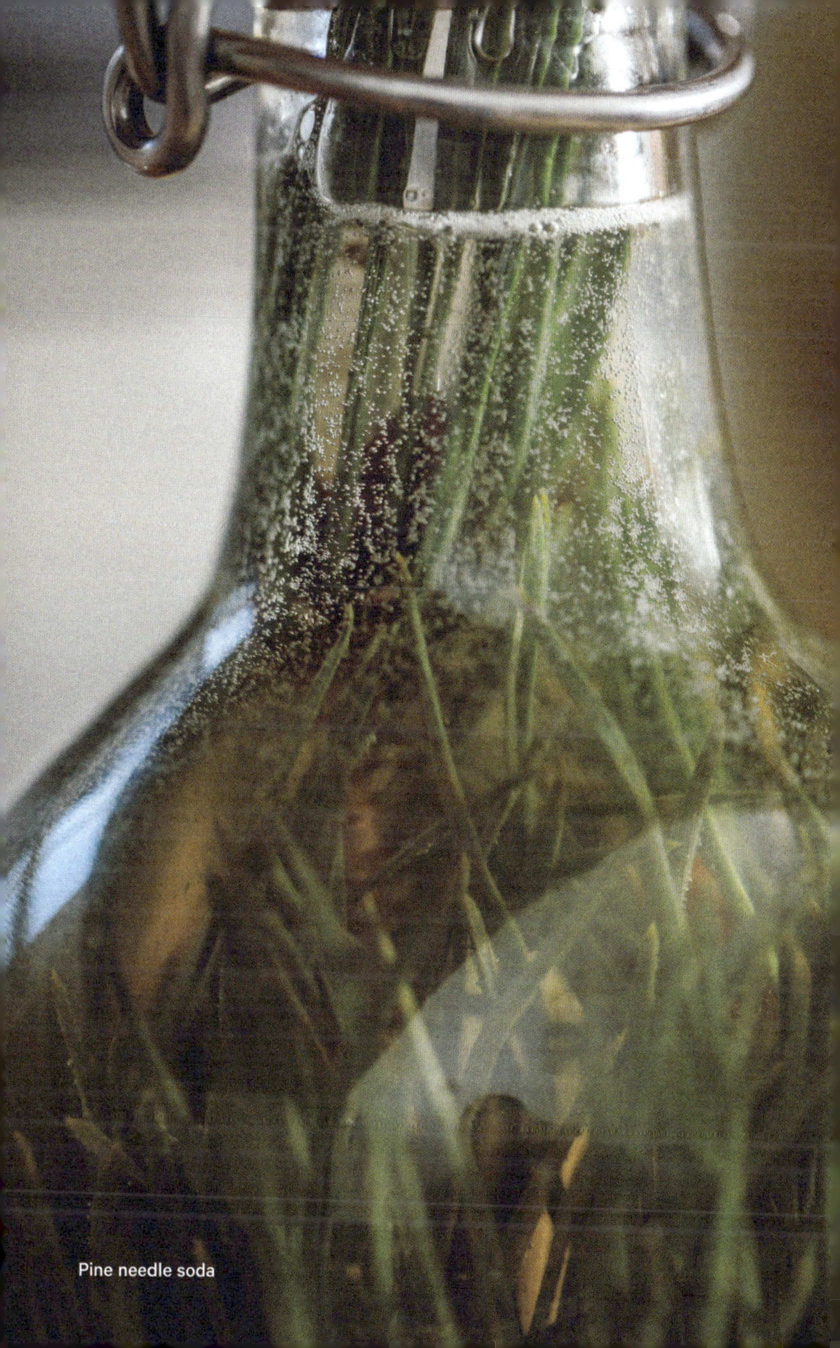

Pine needle soda

with a foraging guide to ensure you have the correct one. Pine needles are long — between 5–12 cm (2–5 in) — and grow in small clusters. One species of pine, the ponderosa pine, has long been believed to be harmful to pregnant women. Some people consider this to be a myth; however, if you are pregnant, we think it is better to steer clear of consuming any pine just to be completely safe.

KIT: *1 litre (34fl oz) clip-top bottle, funnel, sieve, clean piece of muslin*

about 20 pine needle sprigs
950ml (4 cups) water
60g (4 tbsp) sugar (raw cane or golden caster is best)

Inspect your pine needles for insects and remove any critters. Do not wash the needles as this will wash away some of the yeasts needed for fermentation.

Stuff the clean clip-top bottle with the needles, add the sugar using a dry funnel, and pour in the water, leaving about 2 cm (1 in) of headspace at the top. Clip the lid on and shake the bottle to disperse the sugar. Place the bottle on your work surface but out of direct sunlight.

After 3 days, you should see some action and bubbles forming. Pop the lid to release a little gas and to check the status of fermentation. The total time will depend on how many wild yeasts were present and the room temperature. You may need to clip the lid back on and give it another few days until it reaches your desired taste and fizziness. You're aiming for a balance of sweetness, sourness and carbonation. If there's little 'action', move the bottle somewhere slightly warmer — 15–18°C (59–64°F) is optimal.

Your soda should be ready after 7–10 days. Strain through a sieve lined with a piece of muslin into a bottle. If you're not planning to drink it immediately, we advise storing it in a plastic carbonated drinks bottle. If you are against using plastic and want to use the same glass clip-top bottle, just remember to 'burp' it by releasing the lid every 2 days to let gas escape.

Smreka

Smreka is a light, slightly sparkling drink made with juniper berries. Originating from Bosnia, it ferments using the wild yeasts found on the berries and is very simple to make. It takes around a month to fully ferment, so some patience is needed for this one! You can use dried juniper berries; find them in the spice aisle at the supermarket or in bulk at a whole food shop.

Aftercare

Once made, store your smreka in a bottle that can withstand pressure from the carbonation, and keep refrigerated. You can drink it as it is: the flavour will be light, aromatic and slightly citrusy but it makes a great alternative to tonic in a G&T. If you prefer it sweeter, mix with a little honey when serving.

KIT: *500ml (17fl oz) clip-top or screw-top jar, funnel, sieve, bottle or container to store your finished smreka*

200g (7oz) juniper berries
water

Tip the juniper berries into the jar and cover them with water, leaving a small gap at the top. Leave the jar on the kitchen work surface but out of direct sunlight.

If you're using a clip-top jar, 'burp' your smreka every few days to release the pressure. If using a screw-top jar, just screw the cap on loosely to allow gas to escape on its own.

Check your ferment for bubbles that should start to appear within a few days, indicating fermentation is underway. Every few days, shake the jar (ensure the lid is on securely for that part!).

After roughly 3–4 weeks, your smreka should be ready. The berries will all sink to the bottom, which is a good indication, and you can strain into a bottle using a funnel and sieve to store in the fridge.

Kvass

Kvass is a bubbly, sour, fermented drink with Eastern European origins traditionally made using bread. It's a great way of using up your stale bread, and it can be flavoured with a variety of herbs or fruits if you like. This recipe uses a 'kick-starter' to aid the fermentation process, which can be some sourdough starter, kefir water, or dried yeast powder.

KIT: *Saucepan, small plate or lid which just fits inside your pan, 2 clean pieces of muslin, 1–1.5 litre (34–50fl oz) clip-top jar, elastic band, funnel, sieve, clip-top or plastic bottle to store your finished kvass*

—

2 litres (8 cups) water
100g (3½oz) golden caster sugar / unrefined sugar

a few slices of rye or sourdough bread, toasted
kick-starter: 1 tbsp sourdough starter, 3 tbsp water kefir or a pinch of dried yeast powder
a handful of organic (unsulphured) raisins
sprig of herbs such as mint or thyme (optional)

Put the water and sugar into a saucepan and bring to the boil to dissolve the sugar then remove from the heat. Chop the toasted bread into chunks and add it to the sugar solution. Use a lid or plate to weigh the bread pieces down, then let them cool overnight.

Strain the bread mixture into a jug through a sieve lined with a piece of muslin. Twist the muslin corners together to squeeze as much liquid out as possible.

Pour the liquid into a large jar and add your kick-starter plus the raisins and herbs, if using. Give it a mix, then secure the other piece of muslin over the top with the elastic band. Do not use the lid here — you want a bit of airflow. The muslin will keep out any bugs and ensure gas can escape.

Leave the jar at room temperature and out of direct sunlight, ideally at about 15–18°C (59–64°F). After 3–5 days, the mixture should be fizzy and the taste should be a balance of sweet and sour. The longer you leave it, the drier and less sweet it should become. When your kvass reaches your desired taste, strain and bottle it, then leave it on the work surface for 1–2 days to further carbonate. Store in the fridge. If using glass bottles, 'burp' them now and then to release the pressure.

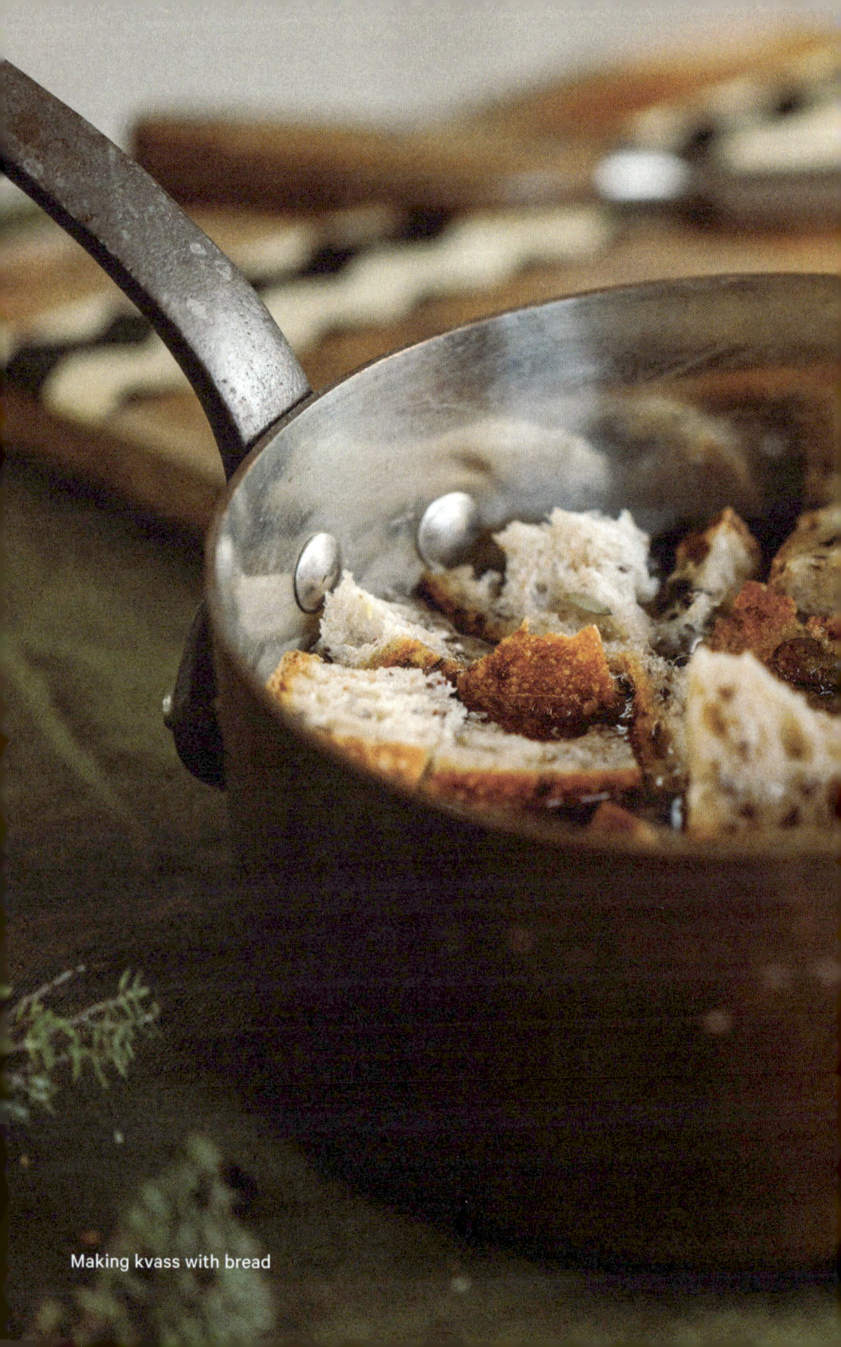
Making kvass with bread

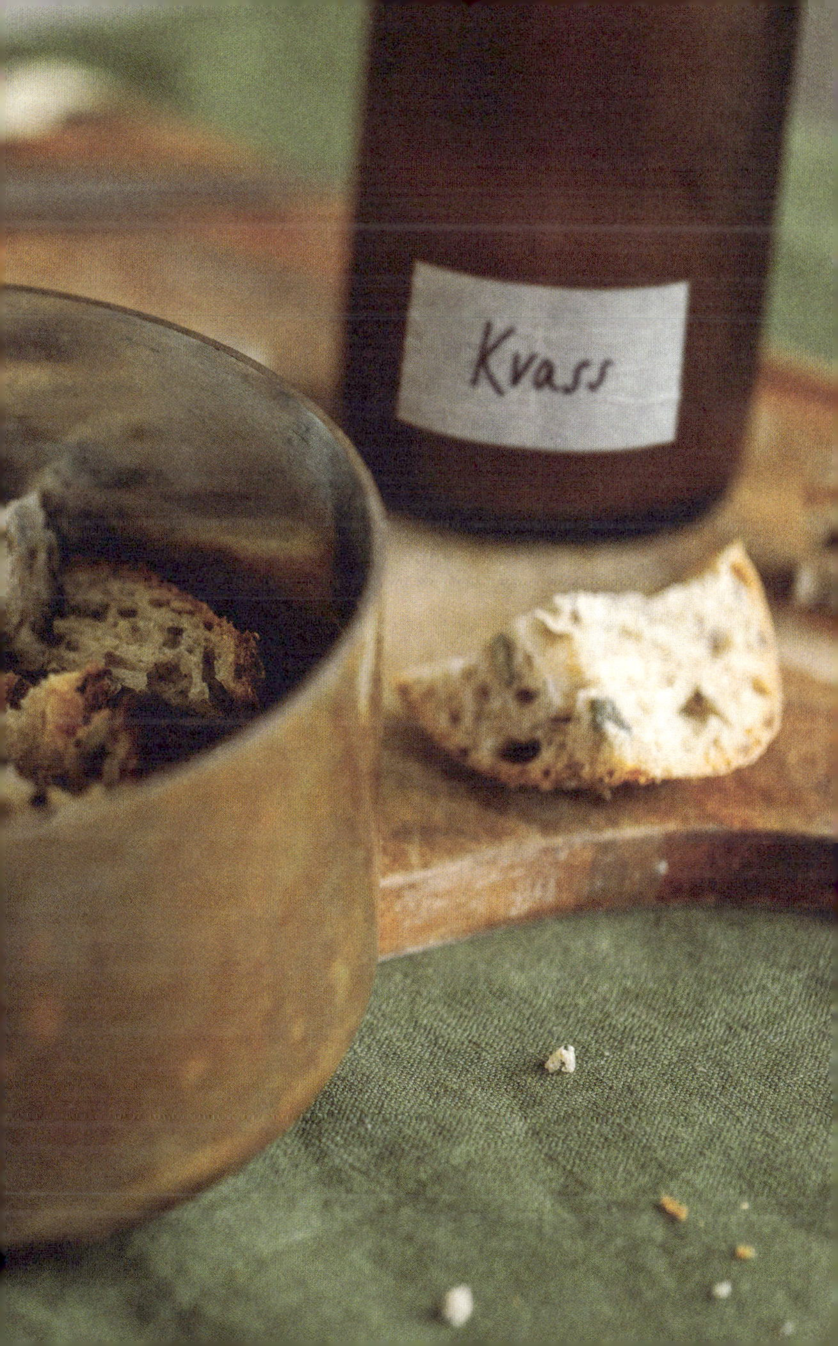
Kvass

Beetroot kvass

This lovely variation of kvass is made using beetroot, which is high in folate, potassium, iron and Vitamin B and produces a wonderfully earthy, naturally sweet sparkling kvass.

Here, we slightly amended the bread kvass recipe, leaving the beetroot pieces in for the whole fermentation process. Once you've strained them, you can use them in a salad.

KIT: *Saucepan, small plate or lid which just fits inside your pan, 2 clean pieces of muslin, 1.5 litre (50fl oz) clip-top jar, elastic band, funnel, sieve, round glass clip-top or plastic carbonated drinks bottle to store*

—

50g (2oz) golden caster sugar / unrefined sugar
1 litre (4 cups) water
2–3 raw beetroots
kick-starter: 1 tbsp sourdough starter, 3 tbsp water kefir or a pinch of dried yeast powder
a handful of organic (unsulphured) raisins
2 star anise, 2 cloves, 1 cinnamon stick (optional)

Put the water and sugar into a saucepan and bring to the boil to dissolve the sugar. Allow it to cool to room temperature. Scrub the beetroots and remove any roots, but do not peel them. Chop them into 1 cm (½ in) chunks and add to the jar, pouring the sugar solution over the top.

Add your kick-starter plus the raisins and spices, if using. Give it a mix, then secure a piece of muslin over the top with the elastic band. Again, do not use the lid here as you want a bit of airflow.

Leave the jar at room temperature and out of direct sunlight, ideally at about 15–18°C (59–64°F). After a couple of days, the mixture should have started to fizz. When your kvass reaches your desired taste (usually after 3–5 days), strain out the beetroot and spices using a funnel and a sieve lined with muslin, bottle it and leave it out on the work surface for a further 1–2 days to carbonate a little more. Store in the fridge. If using clip-top bottles, 'burp' them every now and then to release the pressure.

Mugolio

Mugolio, or fermented pine cone syrup, is traditionally made using green pine cones from the Mugo pine. It requires a slightly longer fermentation, but it is straightforward and gratifying for those with patience! The outcome is a beautifully dark, woody syrup with a slight citrus flavour.

This recipe works well using any edible pine cone — just ensure you have young, green or 'unripe' cones. If they're fingernail-sized, you can keep them whole. Larger cones can be chopped into quarters.

Mugolio can elevate dishes in so many ways. Pour it over ice cream, top crumbles and sweet pies, drizzle it over soft cheeses, or use it to make a cocktail. See pages 146–147 for cocktail recipes we love.

KIT: *Clean jar large enough to fit all your pine cones, glass or plastic bottle / jar for the finished syrup*

—

green pine cones
demerara, light muscovado or raw cane sugar, double the weight of cones that you have

Inspect your pine cones and remove any bugs. Place them in the jar and pour the sugar on top. Screw or clip on the lid and shake the jar to mix the sugar, then leave it somewhere warm to macerate, ideally at 17–21°C (62–70°F).

Shake the jar occasionally to mix the sugar evenly. After a couple of weeks, the cones will release some liquid, and fermentation should have begun. You may see bubbles forming. If your jar has a clip-top lid, burp it once a week to release some gas.

To make a deep and rich pine syrup will take about two months. If you want to preserve this as a culinary syrup for use in the coming weeks, strain the syrup of any pine cones and gently heat it in a pan until it simmers. Bottle it in heatproof glass and refrigerate once cool. Applying heat to near boiling point kills off wild yeasts and pasteurises the syrup. If you leave the syrup unheated, eventually, it will turn into a very dry resinous alcohol, as ours did after a year or so. Nearing year three, our pine spirit is tasting fascinating. This recipe has two potential outcomes, both captivating, and the choice is yours.

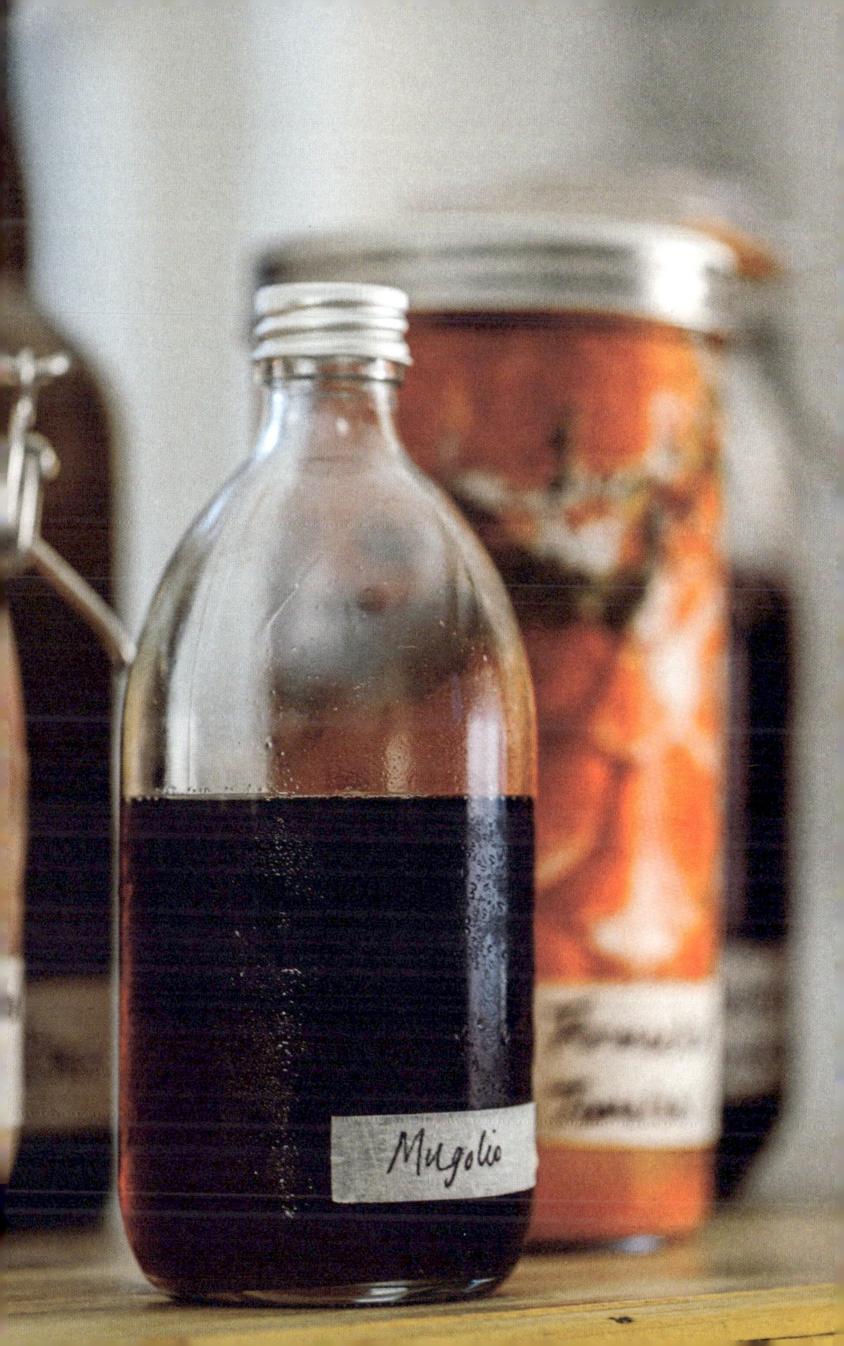
Mugolio

Our cocktail and mocktail recommendations

Gin & water kefir, aka G&WK

50ml (1½fl oz) gin
200ml (scant 1 cup) water kefir

—

Mix over ice, garnish with a slice of lemon.
This is especially good if you have secondary fermented your kefir with fruit such as rhubarb or some berries.

Rum Collins

50ml (1½fl oz) dark rum
25ml (1½ tbsp) lime juice
150ml (⅔ cup) tepache

—

Mix over ice, garnish with basil or mint.
Omit the rum for a mocktail.

Forest Spritz

50ml (1½fl oz) vodka
15ml (1 tbsp) mugolio
a squeeze of lemon juice
150ml (⅔ cup) pine needle soda

—

Shake vodka, mugolio and lemon juice to combine, pour over ice and top with the pine needle soda.
This is another drink that works well as a non-alcoholic version, without the vodka.

Shrub Sour

50ml (1½fl oz) vodka or gin
35ml (1fl oz) shrub
25ml (1½ tbsp) honey
1 egg white

—

Shake all ingredients, then add ice and shake again. Strain to remove the ice and serve in a coupe glass.
We also like this with a non-alcoholic spirit such as Everleaf or Pentire in place of the alcohol.

Mugolio Old Fashioned

50ml (1½fl oz) whisky
15ml (1 tbsp) mugolio
3 dashes of Angostura bitters

—

Gently stir to combine in a whisky tumbler over ice. Garnish with orange peel.

Fermented Bloody Mary

50ml (1½fl oz) vodka
25ml (1½ tbsp) sherry
25ml (1½ tbsp) Worcestershire sauce
50ml (1½fl oz) fermented tomato water
125ml (½ cup) tomato juice
a few dashes of fermented chilli drops

—

Combine in a long glass over ice and garnish with a celery stick.
Leave out the vodka and sherry for a Virgin Mary.

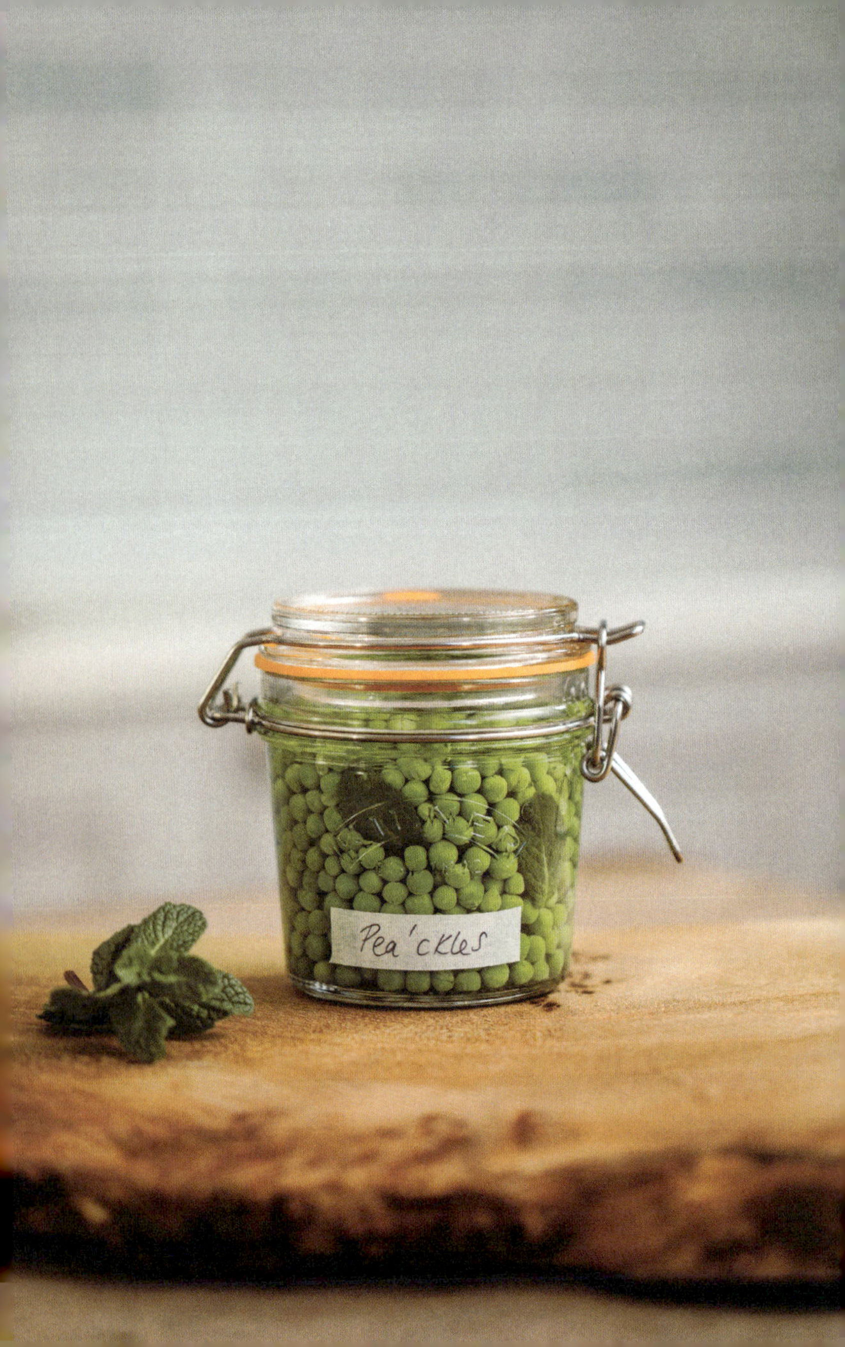
Pea'ckles

Conclusion

By now, you've started to step into the rhythm of food fermentation. You've discovered the science behind it, learned how to preserve seasonal produce and begun to transition away from processed foods. You've found a creative outlet that connects you with nature and the seasons. These skills improve your diet and foster a more mindful relationship with food.

You've gained the ability to recognise the stage of your ferment, troubleshoot any issues that may arise and balance flavour with herbs, spices and botanicals.

You've learned how to pair dishes with your homemade ferments, and by now, you'll have a colourful and enticing larder of gut-nourishing foods and drinks to wow your dinner guests and elevate your meals.

Fermentation is a lifestyle. By incorporating these techniques into your routine, you've embraced a healthier, more sustainable way of living. The journey doesn't end here — continue exploring, experimenting and sharing your delicious creations.

Thank you for joining us in this journey of curiosity and understanding. We hope *Do Ferment* has inspired you to make fermentation a joyful and integral part of your life. Here's to a future filled with nutritious, flavourful ferments!

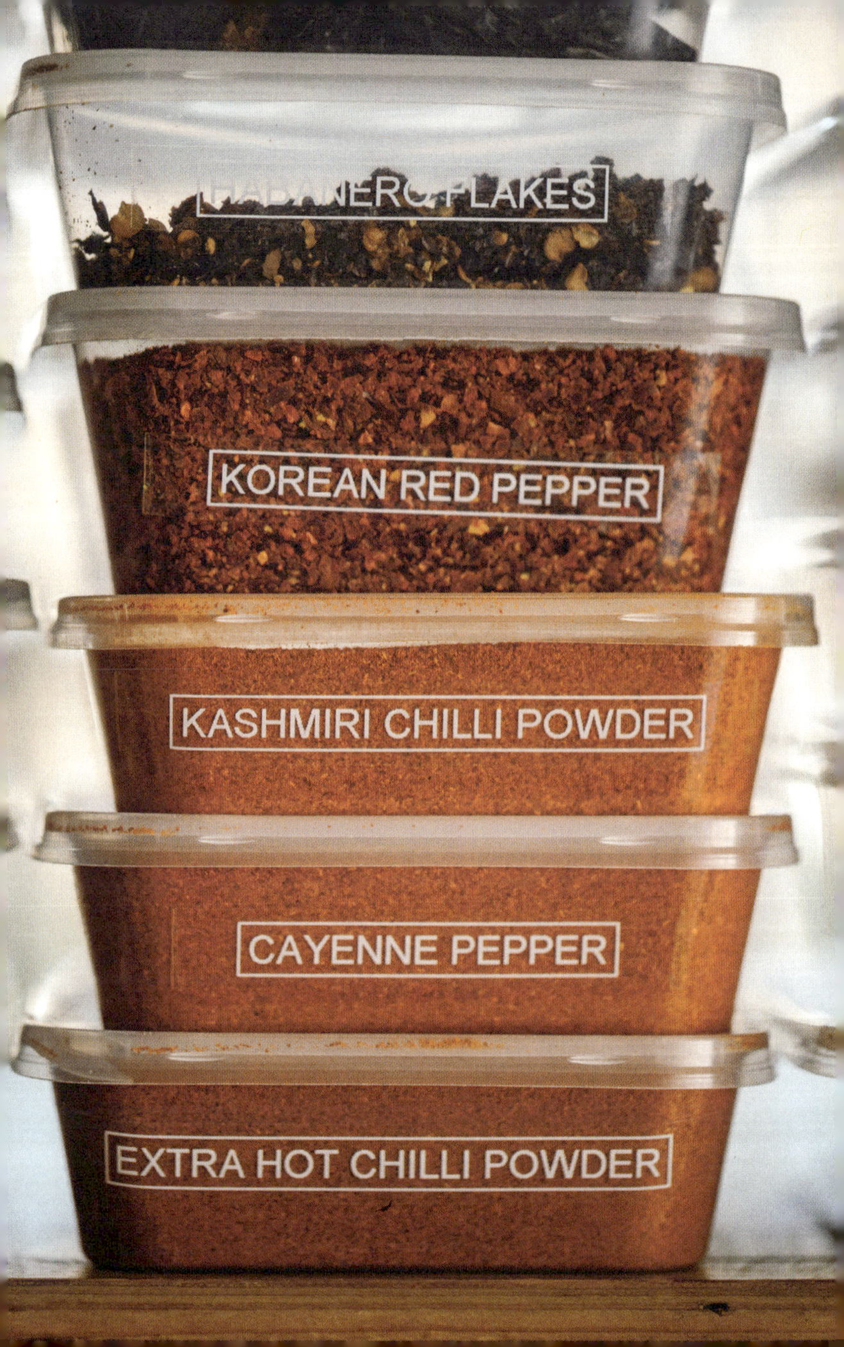
HABANERO FLAKES
KOREAN RED PEPPER
KASHMIRI CHILLI POWDER
CAYENNE PEPPER
EXTRA HOT CHILLI POWDER

Resources

Books and guides

Mentioned in the book
On Food and Cooking
by Harold McGee
Immune
by Philipp Dettmer
The Flavour Thesaurus
by Niki Segnit

Pine foraging identification
conifers.fscbiodiversity.uk

Foraging wild garlic
Edible and Medicinal Wild Plants of Britain and Ireland
by Robin Harford

Suppliers

Jars
kilnerjar.co.uk
kilnerjar.com
ballmasonjars.com

pH testers
happykombucha.co.uk

Salt
halenmon.com
blackthornsalt.co.uk
redmond.life

Kefir grains
everygoodthing.co.uk
freshlyfermented.co.uk
happykombucha.co.uk
culturesforhealth.com

Spices
buywholefoodsonline.co.uk
souschef.co.uk

About the authors

Matthew Pennington With a career in food that began at the age of 15, Matthew has embarked on a journey of exploration that has profoundly shaped his worldview. Combining interests in cooking, native produce, wild food, fermentation, regenerative agriculture, soil health, mycology, tradition, food folklore and philosophy, Matthew has dedicated his career to pursuing culinary crafts connected to nature.

He is a published author and has appeared on television to advocate for food fermentation, soil health and regenerative food systems. His restaurant project, The Ethicurean, held prestigious awards for its environmental approach and culinary consideration.

Self-taught, Matthew believes the kitchen and garden can unlock almost any subject, from the sciences to the philosophical. He is happiest sharing his knowledge at a table filled with food, friends and curiosity.

Nicola Cradock Nicola's love of food and drink took root in childhood as she grew up on her family's fourth-generation farm in Wiltshire. She learned to appreciate the rhythms of nature and the connection between land, food and community—values that continue to shape her approach to living and working sustainably.

Her passion lies in the alchemy of fermentation, particularly with drinks. Since joining Matthew at his restaurant in 2017, she has delved into crafting wild sparkling sodas, fruit wines and kefirs, always chasing depth of flavour and new flavour combinations. The slow, hands-on processes bring moments of stillness to her busy days, and she takes delight in sharing her creations—bottled, fizzing and full of life—with friends and family around her.

Nicola and Matthew live in Edinburgh with their lurcher, Lint. They are working on a platform centred around reconnecting with nature, building community and transforming people's relationship with food.

They teach classes in fermentation, foraging and cooking across the UK, offer private dining, and consult with like-minded, forward-thinking and responsible businesses.

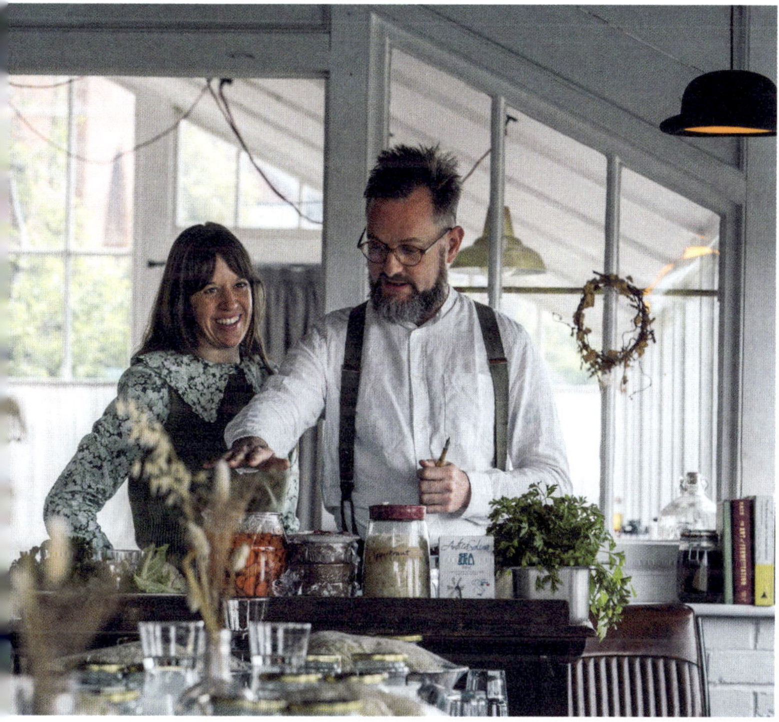

Thanks

Family

Where we lean, where we learn, where we love.

To our beloved family, you've held us with warmth to fizz, and just the right amount of salt to keep us balanced. Your encouragement, support and love has lifted us and given us the confidence to find purpose and 'Do'. To the Cradocks — Joanne and Ian, Benjy, Ashley, Aimee, Jess, Sue and Steve, Grampy, Pauline, Sandra; and the Penningtons — John and Janey, Tara, Ellie, Iain, Molly, Dan, Emma Noble and the Lawtons — we are endlessly grateful.

Do team

Miranda, Jess and the Do Books team — your support, enthusiasm and brilliant minds have shaped this book in ways we're truly grateful for. To David Hieatt and the DO Lectures — thank you for creating a space where ideas grow wild and take root and for bringing us into the fold.

Photoshoot

Remco Merbis, for capturing the detail of our world with such beauty. Polishka, Matt and Sonia, your generosity brought the vision. Kilner, for the jars that hold our bubbling ideas. Twelve Triangles Portobello, for furnishing us with pastries, sourdough and props.

Friends

To the friends who have cheered us on: Polishka, Leanne and Jim, Jude and Matt, Sonia and Matt, Angela and Tim, Simon Miller, Mark, Peter, Michelle, Martin Maudsley, Rob and Keir, Sandy and Jane, Martin and Jin, Amy and Si, Mandy, Daisy, Gem, Emma, Joanna. You've been our partners in brine and, most importantly, our people.

Inspirational producers

To every grower, regenerative farmer, and, of course, the blessed cheesemakers. Hodmedod's, for proving that the future is in the soil. Halen Môn, for reminding us that salt is life. The Free Company, for showing that regenerative food, farm to fork and community are inseparable.

Authors

Niki Segnit, Benjamin Hoff, Robin Harford, Harold McGee —your words have sparked ideas, deepened our curiosity and reminded us why we do what we do.

The Ethicurean Restaurant

To Iain and Mark, thank you for exploring the art of fermentation with us and bringing the restaurant to its finest iteration. To every Ethicurean team ambassador, customer, and producer—thank you for being part of something in another realm.

To Mark Cox, for tending a living garden like no other and countless moments of utmost deliciousness.

To our ferment class attendees – your curiosity and enthusiasm keep the culture alive.

To Paûla and Jack, thank you for shaping the early years.

You and those who do

If these pages have found their way to you, we hope they inspire, guide and encourage you to get your hands in the brine, embrace the process and share the joy.

With gratitude and a good pinch of salt,
Nicola & Matthew

Index

Books in the series

Do Agile Tim Drake
Do Beekeeping Orren Fox
Do Birth Caroline Flint
Do Bitcoin Angelo Morgan-Somers
Do Blue Nick Hounsfield & Abby Richardson
Do Breathe Michael Townsend Williams
Do Build Alan Moore
Do Conversation Robert Poynton
Do Deal Richard Hoare & Andrew Gummer
Do Death Amanda Blainey
Do Design Alan Moore
Do Disrupt Mark Shayler
Do Drama Lucy Gannon
Do Earth Tam Omond
Do Ferment Matthew Pennington & Nicola Cradock
Do Fly Gavin Strange
Do Grow Alice Holden
Do Hope Gail Muller
Do Improvise Robert Poynton
Do Inhabit Sue Fan & Danielle Quigley
Do Interesting Russell Davies
Do Lead Les McKeown
Do Listen Bobette Buster
Do Loss Sue Deagle
Do Maintain Gareth Heaton
Do Make James Otter
Do Nourish Sarah Bayliss
Do Open David Hieatt
Do Pause Robert Poynton
Do Photo Andrew Paynter
Do Present Mark Shayler
Do Preserve Anja Dunk, Jen Goss & Mimi Beaven
Do Protect Johnathan Rees
Do Purpose David Hieatt
Do Recruit Khalilah Olokunola
Do Reset Jillian Lavender
Do Scale Les McKeown
Do Sea Salt Alison, David & Jess Lea-Wilson
Do Sing James Sills
Do Smoke Jen Goss & Scott Davis
Do Sourdough Andrew Whitley
Do Start Dan Kieran
Do Story Bobette Buster
Do Team Charlie Gladstone
Do Walk Libby DeLana
Do Wild Baking Tom Herbert

Also available

The Book of Do ed. Miranda West
Path Louisa Thomsen Brits
The Skimming Stone Dominic Wilcox
Stay Curious Clare Hieatt
The Path of a Doer David Hieatt

DO Book Co

Available in print, digital and audio formats from booksellers or via our website: **thedobook.co**. To hear about events and forthcoming titles, find us on social media **@dobookco**, or subscribe to our newsletter.